Essentials of Nursing Research

ABOUT THE AUTHOR

Lucille E. Notter, R.N., Ed.D., until very recently the editor of *Nursing Research* as well as the *International Nursing Index,* and project director of the American Nurses' Association Annual Nursing Research Conferences (1965–1973), draws on a wide background in nursing, including staff nursing, supervision, nursing education, administration, and public health nursing. She has served on many local, state, and national boards and committees, both lay and professional. Dr. Notter has published extensively in leading nursing journals and is the co-author, with Eugenia K. Spalding, of *Professional Nursing: Foundations, Perspectives and Relationships.* Currently, Dr. Notter is co-editor of *Cardiovascular Nursing.*

Essentials of Nursing Research

LUCILLE E. NOTTER

SPRINGER PUBLISHING COMPANY, INC.
New York

To my friend

Jane D. Keeler

*for her unfailing encourage-
ment and support during my
various attempts at writing
—including the preparation
of this book*

SPRINGER PUBLISHING COMPANY, INC.
200 Park Avenue South, New York, New York 10003

Library of Congress Catalog Card Number: 73-88107
International Standard Book Number: 0-8261-1590-X

77 78 / 10 9 8 7 6

Acknowledgement: The ratio for the *t* test on p. 92 is reprinted by permission of the author and publisher from
Better Patient Care through Nursing Research, by Faye
G. Abdellah and Eugene Levine (New York: Macmillan,
1965). © copyright, The Macmillan Company, 1965.

Printed in U.S.A.

CONTENTS

v

FOREWORD

Increasingly with each decade, greater numbers of nurses are becoming involved in the research of their profession. Also, the rudiments of the research process are now being introduced at the undergraduate level, whereas in the past research experience was almost entirely limited to graduate education in nursing. It seems strange that as greater numbers of nurses are being prepared at the doctoral level in research methodology, the end result does not reflect more postgraduate nursing research activity. Perhaps this may be attributed in part to the attitude toward research that has been inculcated in nurses during their educational experiences, and in part to the complexity of approach and the overwhelming statistical methods which are used in most textbooks on research and which serve to discourage nurses from undertaking research studies.

Historically, textbooks and guidelines for the conduct of nursing research have relied upon other disciplines, especially the social sciences, for research approaches. Very few basic guides for research in nursing, particularly for clinical nursing, exist. Consequently, Dr. Notter's *Essentials of Nursing Research* is an important contribution. This book gives the beginning researcher, whether she is an undergraduate or a graduate nursing student, a relatively simple, progressive, and comprehensive guide to follow. The development of the book logically follows the steps in the research process from the investigator's first spark of an idea through to the communication of the results of a study. The information is presented in a clear, straightforward, and interesting manner, and is well documented with examples of clinical studies in nursing. This text should help to establish a healthy respect for nursing research and stimulate interest in it among practitioners and students alike.

Phyllis J. Verhonick

ACKNOWLEDGMENTS

The author wishes to express her deep appreciation for the significant influence of many professional colleagues who, over the years, have contributed to the enrichment of her professional experience and made the writing of this book possible. A special vote of thanks goes to Mary Ann Garrigan, professor of nursing and curator of the Nursing Archive of the Mugar Memorial Library at Boston University, for first suggesting this basic guide to nursing research and to Helen Behnke, whose excellent suggestions and patient editing are deeply appreciated. Joan Sanger, copy editor of *Nursing Research,* made valuable editorial suggestions regarding the final manuscript. Finally, the author wishes to thank the American Journal of Nursing Company for allowing her to use certain copyrighted materials, particularly from the journal *Nursing Research.*

PREFACE

Every nurse has a part to play in nursing research, whether it be participation in research itself or as a user of the products of research. Thus, the research nurse and the practitioner have a common goal—to provide the best nursing care possible. Research can help us find scientific answers to problems in nursing which, in turn, can result in the achievement of this goal, provided that researchers and practitioners join forces.

Clinical studies (called applied research) aimed at improved practice and better patient care, as well as basic research aimed at expanding the frontiers of knowledge, have been proposed to meet the need for the development and testing of nursing theories. Although an increasing number of specially qualified nurses are engaged in both clinical and basic research, it is important for all nurses to be aware of this need and to participate to the extent that they can.

Practitioners can participate in research in many ways. They can keep abreast of the new knowledge coming out of research, identify clinical problems for which research is needed and communicate this need to researchers, cooperate when research projects are initiated in their institutions, and assist in research projects as data collectors. In addition, many young practitioners are beginning to be interested in doing research themselves and are seeking help in developing the skills required to carry out simple but carefully designed studies in the clinical setting. Some institutions now employ research consultants whose function is to stimulate and guide nurses in the conduct of such studies. These small, less sophisticated

studies, which have been called "research with a small *r*," *
will be done by many nurses with only elementary skills in
research — practitioners and clinicians whose intellectual
curiosity and spirit of inquiry lead them to observe problems
at first hand, define them, and begin to study them. The
results of their efforts may inspire more comprehensive,
sophisticated studies of the additional problems or questions
they bring to light.

Eventually, the findings of research must be applied in
practice if they are to effect improvement in patient care. This
goal can be achieved only if practicing nurses are aware of
research projects being carried out and can read and evaluate
the findings in terms of their implications for nursing care.
Research-oriented nurses will be able to make the most effective use of the findings of research in their daily practice.

To write about so complex a process as scientific research
so that the result will be useful to undergraduate students of
nursing and to graduates who have had little prior preparation
in research methods may pose difficulties. Nevertheless, I
believe that many nurses are indeed interested in learning some
basic facts about research, about how to evaluate its usefulness
for them, and about how they can become participants in
nursing research. Therefore, I have tried to present the facts
simply and concisely for this particular audience. If this book
serves to help nurses and nursing in these ways, my purpose
in writing it will have been satisfied.

Lucille E. Notter

*See Ramshorn, Mary T. Small *r* in nursing research: an exploratory study of patient experiences in isolation. *J N Y State Nurses'
Assn* 3:24-29, Dec. 1972.

I

INTRODUCTION
TO RESEARCH

1

EVOLUTION OF THE RESEARCH MOVEMENT IN NURSING

From the beginning of time men have raised questions about their experiences and the nature of activities going on around them and have looked for answers that would help them understand and deal with problems they encountered. Nurses have become interested in research because they too want to find answers to questions that trouble them—scientific answers. All kinds of nurses in many kinds of situations have raised questions about themselves, their education, and their practice.

Historically, four main approaches have been used to explain phenomena: magic, authority, logical reasoning, and the scientific method. Over the years nurses have used all these approaches to explain activities or solve problems.

Primitive man relied upon magic or the influence of some supernatural power for an explanation of facts that he could not understand. Later, wise men or authorities were consulted to provide the answers that were needed. Because of their experience, or their ability to think through problems and formulate answers, they were counted on to give valid opinions. Authorities, or experts, continue to be used. This is legitimate practice in many instances—at times because answers are needed immediately and there is no time for research, and at times because the resources or tools needed to do the required

3

research are not available. It must be remembered, however, that authorities may not always give the best answers and, on occasion, they may give incomplete or even wrong answers.

Logical reasoning, which ancient Greek civilization employed to such advantage, provided a mental tool for examining the universe and man's behavior. Logic, which is basic to the scientific method, involves inductive and deductive reasoning. The Greek contribution to scientific thinking was primarily the use of deductive reasoning, that is, the development of logical answers or conclusions from reliable premises. Of course, in deductive reasoning a great deal depends on the soundness of the premise. Inductive reasoning explains relationships by obtaining facts through observation and making generalizations based upon these facts.

Scientific method, or research as we know it today, has been in use for a relatively short period of time, approximately 300 years. It makes use of logical reasoning; for example, the hypotheses to be tested by research, the methods of research used, and the conclusions reached as a result of research must always be logical.

Modern research, or scientific inquiry, may also make use of experts, or authorites. Ideas or generalizations to be tested may be obtained from the experts as well as from practitioners. However, scientific inquiry provides a method whereby our ideas, hunches, or hypotheses can be systematically tested and valid evidence about the truth of the matter can be obtained. It rejects reliance upon chance or magic, trial and error, or generalizations based on reasoning and experience alone.

RESEARCH IN NURSING

Since nursing is a practice profession, nurses have, in the past, placed more emphasis on its practical aspects than on research. Thus, nurses tended to accept ideas and knowledge from authorities without much question.

Unlike many other professions, nursing was slow to develop the partnership between practitioner and investigator which is so necessary to achieve progress toward the ultimate goal—in this case, improved nursing care. There are several reasons for this situation. First, despite her skill in scientific investigation, Florence Nightingale laid the foundation for modern nursing education within the framework of the military tradition, which emphasizes the concept of authority. Schools of nursing that developed in hospitals throughout the world, including the United States, were strongly influenced by the British pattern of nursing education and thus continued to foster reliance upon tradition and authority. It is interesting to speculate what might have happened had Miss Nightingale encouraged the spirit of inquiry in nursing as she did in other fields.

In a discussion of the development of research in nursing, Simmons and Henderson (1964, p. 7) pointed out that the development of research within the established professions, and the wealth of knowledge these professions have generated in the brief span of time that modern research methods have been used, are directly related to the development of formal education within the university, a setting that serves as a center for research and research training. These authors suggested that it was necessary for nursing education programs to be established within universities—a fairly recent development —before nurses could be prepared to do research. They also pointed to the fact that nursing education was influenced by the general status of all women in this country and by the education facilities available to women prior to the turn of the century. University education for women then was certainly far from the common occurrence it is today.

EARLY DAYS OF NURSING RESEARCH
IN THE UNITED STATES

As nursing developed in this country, leadership resided primarily in the educators who operated under the strong belief that nursing practice would be improved through improvement in the quality of nursing education. This thesis was logical in the light of the status of nursing education, which was primarily an apprenticeship, and the status of education of women generally. These nursing educators were often responsible not only for the administration of the school but also for the nursing service. As a result, during the first half of this century research in nursing in this country was directed more toward improved education or nursing service administration rather than toward improved practice.

M. Adelaide Nutting's survey of nursing education, published in 1906, was probably the earliest important study done by an American nurse. A few studies by nurses aimed at improving nursing care appeared in the literature in the 1920s and 1930s. These nurse authors were most often concerned with studies of nursing procedures or with time studies. Broadhurst et al. (1927) studied hand brushing, Wasserberg and Northam (1927) did a time study in obstetrical nursing, Cowan (1929) carried out a comparative study of two methods of breast care, Pfefferkorn (1932) described time studies, Ryan and Miller (1932) did a thermometer study, and, finally, Wheeler (1938) reported on her study of tuberculosis nursing care.

Of considerable influence in promoting nursing studies during this period were persons like Isabel Stewart and Mary M. Marvin. In 1927 Marvin made a plea in the *American Journal of Nursing* for nursing experimentation. She stated that there were:

> six phases of experimentation which would help us in developing practical nursing along safer, sounder lines: First, an exhaustive study of nursing procedures from the standpoint of the biological and physical sciences; second, an analysis of nursing procedures on the basis of elimination of waste in materials, cost, energy, etc.; third, a comparative study of all equipment and materials used in the care of the sick; fourth, experimentation to find better methods of teaching the subject; fifth, tests for vocational aptitudes before the students enter the school; and sixth, tests of nursing performance, to determine the skill attained at any stage of teaching (pp. 331–332).

As we can see, half of her suggestions focused upon studies of nursing procedures; the others were related to educational research. Nevertheless, interest in clinically oriented research was beginning, although few nurses at that time were qualified to do research. Nursing research done in the 1930s and 1940s was frequently carried out by persons from other disciplines. Two well-known examples of such studies were Esther Lucile Brown's *Nursing for the Future* (1948) and *A Program for the Nursing Profession* (1948) by the Committee on the Function of Nursing, chaired by Eli Ginsberg.

NURSING RESEARCH IN THE 1950s AND 1960s

Research as a major movement in nursing received its first effective impetus in the 1950s. As a result of the recommendations of the Brown (1948) and Bridgman (1953) studies, among other developments, emphasis on baccalaureate and graduate education for nurses increased. Masters programs for nurses were developing and a growing number of nurses were going on for the doctoral degree.

Some of the activities of the 1950s that influenced the development of nursing research were:

1. *1950.* The House of Delegates of the American Nurses' Association voted to initiate a nationwide program of studies of nursing functions. Several state and local nursing groups were involved in the program, which was reported in *Nurses Invest in Patient Care* (American Nurses' Association, 1956) and in *Twenty Thousand Nurses Tell Their Story* (Hughes et al., 1958).

2. *1952.* Through the efforts of the Association of Collegiate Schools of Nursing, which became part of the National League for Nursing in 1952 (Biennial Highlights, pp. 824-825), the American Journal of Nursing Company began the publication of *Nursing Research.* The purposes of the new journal were: "To inform members of the nursing profession and allied professions of the results of scientific studies in nursing, and to stimulate research in nursing" *(Nursing Research,* Editorial, 1952, p. 5).

3. *1953.* The Institute of Research and Service in Nursing Education was launched at Teachers College, Columbia University (Bunge, 1958), to strengthen and improve education for nursing by conducting research on nursing and nursing education problems and disseminating the results, and by preparing nurses to do research.

4. *1955.* The American Nurses' Association established the American Nurses' Foundation as an independent organization for the purpose of furthering research in nursing by conducting and supporting research projects (Hardin, 1957; Taylor, 1970).

5. *1955.* A Research Grant and Fellowship Branch was set up within the Division of Nursing Resources of the U.S. Public Health Service. Since its establishment, funds have been available for research in nursing, workshops and conferences, faculty development in research methods, fellowships, and nurse scientist training programs (Vreeland, 1964; Abdellah, 1970).

6. *1957.* A Department of Nursing was established within the Walter Reed Army Institute (Werley, 1962). Other federal agencies now have research programs in nursing.

7. *1958.* The House of Delegates of the American Nurses' Association accepted Goal One, which was designed to stimulate nurses and other specialists to identify nursing principles and to do research on the application of these principles (American Nurses' Association, 1960, p. 146). The Association's Committee on Research and Studies was given responsibility for planning activities related to this research goal. They recognized two main activities: development of a corps of nurse researchers and development of intellectual curiosity and critical inquiry in students and in nurse practitioners (American Nurses' Association, 1960). A conference group for nurses qualified in research was formed at the 1958 convention.

Throughout this period, nursing continued to be studied mostly by persons outside the profession. Nurses became one of the most frequently studied occupational groups, chiefly by behavioral scientists, but the study of nursing practice was still largely neglected. By 1959, however, the number of nurses with doctoral degrees reached 151 (Simmons and Henderson, 1964, p. 135), and the number of studies by nurses reported in the literature was evidence of increased emphasis on research in nursing.

The real impetus for research in clinical practice began in the 1960s. Gradually, interest in clinical investigations reported by nurses increased. Often these reports were based on doctoral studies, masters theses, or even occasionally on undergraduate work. Clinical research continued to lag behind other types of studies, however, even though 19 of the 72 articles published by *Nursing Research* in 1969 were related to nursing practice (Notter, 1970). Examples of more recent clinical research studies can be seen in later issues of that journal. For instance, the May-June 1972 issue contained articles by Lindeman, Porter, Verhonick et al., Williams, Nichols et al., and Marshall and Feeney, that reported clinical nursing studies.

NURSING RESEARCH TODAY

Today, preparation in research techniques is an integral part of all graduate study for nurses, and an introduction to research has been made part of undergraduate programs (Verhonick, 1971). As a true partnership develops between researcher and practitioner, nurses will move closer to their common goal—the achievement of better nursing care for patients, care that is based on validated scientific inquiry.

REFERENCES

Abdellah, Faye G. Overview of nursing research 1955–1968. Part I, *Nurs Res* 19:6–17, Jan.-Feb. 1970; Part II, *Nurs Res* 19:151–162, Mar.-Apr. 1970; and Part III, *Nurs Res* 19:239–252, May-June 1970.

American Nurses' Association. *House of Delegates Reports, 1958–1960.* New York, The Association, 1960.

————. *Nurses Invest in Patient Care.* New York, The Association, 1956.

Biennial Highlights. *Am J Nurs* 52:824–827, July 1952.

Bridgman, Margaret. *Collegiate Education for Nursing.* New York, Russell Sage Foundation, 1953.

Broadhurst, Jean; Rang, Geraldine G.; and Schoening, Elsa. Hand brush suggestions for visiting nurses. *Public Health Nurs* 19:487–489, Oct. 1927.

Brown, Esther Lucile. *Nursing for the Future.* New York, Russell Sage Foundation, 1948.

Bunge, Helen L. The Institute of Research and Service in Nursing Education, Teachers College, Columbia University. *Nurs Res* 7:113–115, Oct. 1958.

Committee on the Function of Nursing (Eli Ginsberg, Chairman). *A Program for the Nursing Profession.* New York, Macmillan, 1948.

Cowan, Cordelia M. A study of breast care. Part I, *Am J Nurs* 29:1165–1170, Oct. 1929; Part II, *Am J Nurs* 29:1299–1306, Nov. 1929.

Editorial. A cooperative venture. *Nurs Res* 1:5, June 1952.

Hardin, Clara. The American Nurses' Foundation builds a program. *Am J Nurs* 57:310–311, Mar. 1957.

Hughes, Everett C.; Hughes, Helen MacGill; and Deutscher, Irwin. *Twenty Thousand Nurses Tell Their Story.* Philadelphia, J. B. Lippincott, 1958.

Lindeman, Carol A. Nursing intervention with the presurgical patient: effectiveness and efficiency of group and individual preoperative teaching—Phase II. *Nurs Res* 21:196–209, May-June 1972.

Marshall, Jon C. and Feeney, Sally. Structured versus intuitive intake interview. *Nurs Res* 21:269–272, May-June 1972.

Marvin, Mary M. Research in nursing. *Am J Nurs* 27:331–335, May 1927.

Nichols, Glennadee A.; Kulvi, Ruth L.; Life, Hazel R.; and Christ, Nancy M. Measuring oral and rectal temperatures of febrile children. *Nurs Res* 21:261–264, May-June 1972.

Notter, Lucille E. Report of the editor—1970. (editorial) *Nurs Res* 19:5, Jan.-Feb. 1970.

Nutting, M. Adelaide. The education and professional position of nurses. In *Report of the Commissioner of Education for the Year Ending June 30, 1906.* Washington, D.C., Government Printing Office, 1907, pp. 155–205.

Pfefferkorn, Blanche. Measuring nursing, quantitatively and qualitatively. *Am J Nurs* 32:80–84, Jan. 1932.

Porter, Luz S. The impact of physical-physiological activity on infants' growth and development. *Nurs Res* 21:210–219, May-June 1972.

Ryan, Elizabeth and Miller, Virginia B. Disinfection of clinical thermometers. *Am J Nurs* 32:197–206, Feb. 1932.

Simmons, Leo W. and Henderson, Virginia. *Nursing Research: A Survey and Assessment.* New York, Appleton-Century-Crofts, 1964.

Taylor, Susan D. American Nurses' Foundation, 1955–1970. *Nurs Res Rep* 5:1–6, Dec. 1970.

Verhonick, Phyllis J. Research awareness at the undergraduate level. *Nurs Res* 20:261–265, May-June 1971.

Verhonick, Phyllis J.; Lewis, David W.; and Goller, Herbert O. Thermography in the study of decubitus ulcers. *Nurs Res* 21:233–237, May-June 1972.

Vreeland, Ellwynne M. Nursing research programs of the Public Health Service: highlights and trends. *Nurs Res* 13:148–158, Spring 1964.

Wasserberg, Chelly and Northam, Ethel. Some time studies in obstetrical nursing. *Am J Nurs* 27:543–544, July 1927.

Werley, Harriet H. Promoting the research dimension in the practice of nursing through the establishment and development of a Department of Nursing in an Institute of Research. *Milit Med* 127:219–231, Mar. 1962.

Wheeler, Claribel A. (Ed.) A study of the nursing care of tuberculosis patients. *Am J Nurs* 38:1021–1037, Sept. 1938.

Williams, Anne. A study of factors contributing to skin breakdown. *Nurs Res* 21:238–243, May-June 1972.

2

THE MEANING AND
PURPOSE OF RESEARCH

Why research? And particularly, Why research in nursing? Scientific investigations can be long and costly and may end up with negative findings. However, research, some of which did not at the time appear to have immediate practical value, has been responsible for most of the major advances our society has made in the last century—advances in communication, transportation, agriculture, and the control and treatment of disease, to mention but a few. Modern technology is a direct product of research. Modern medical treatment had its origin in various types of chemical and biological research, both basic and applied. Such simple, taken-for-granted things as refrigeration, air conditioning, radio, and television all came about as a result of the investigations of many scientists. It is easy to see the importance of research in our lives, if we but stop and think about it for a moment.

But what about research in nursing? Is it really needed? Is it really important? In the past, nursing relied heavily on facts and knowledge obtained from authorities, that is, facts and knowledge derived from the experience of experts. It also borrowed facts from other sciences without necessarily testing them scientifically to determine how well they might serve in their new role.

Modern research methods are tools which nurses can employ in studying their practice to obtain scientific evidence needed for validating that practice and for using the findings of their investigations in their practice. Because these methods are known, it would seem that all nurses are morally responsible to use them for the improvement of patient care.

You, as a nurse, can participate in research in several ways. First, you can observe nursing care that is being given and the responses of patients to that care. You can raise questions that should be studied. For example, one nurse observed the incidence of phlebitis in patients with indwelling venous catheters and decided that there might be a relationship between the size and material of the catheter and other selected factors that favor thrombosis such as changes in blood flow, changes in the vein wall, and changes in the clotting mechanism (Ross, 1972). This nurse's exploratory study brought a number of recommendations for further studies. As a result of your observations, you too may undertake an exploratory study, or you may communicate your observations to a nurse researcher who may carry out the study or assist you in doing so. You might think about this and compile a list of observations you would like to make and some of the *variables* that would be involved.*

A second way of participating in nursing research is to assist in the collection of data for a research project. As the amount of nursing research increases, so do the opportunities for nurses to become involved in research programs. Some researchers employ research assistants to help with such data

---

*Just as you needed to learn a new vocabulary in order to become a nurse, so you will need to become familiar with the terminology of research. Throughout this book, research terms are italicized and usually defined the first time they are used. In addition, all these terms are defined in the glossary at the end of this book.

collection procedures as making observations or conducting interviews. Being involved in an investigation and then waiting to see how it turns out, knowing that you have contributed to the project, is an exciting experience.

Being a member of a research team, intra- or inter-disciplinary, is another way of participating. The team may consist of nurses only; for example, the study "Comparison of Three Bowel Management Programs during Rehabilitation of Spinal Cord Injured Patients" was carried out by six nurses (Cornell et al., 1973). On the other hand, you may be the only nurse on a clinical team headed by a sociologist, psychologist, physician, or physiologist. In this case, as the nursing expert, your clinical knowledge will be as important as your knowledge of study methods. You may also, as a team member, be responsible for carrying out an individual piece of research on your own while others on the team are contributing other pieces.

Of course, a principal way of participating in nursing research is to do a study yourself. This book presents some of the basic facts you will need to know before you try even a simple study. In addition, you may want to obtain help from an expert in research—your teacher or a consultant, for example. Your institution may have on its staff a nurse who is qualified in research methods and who is available to assist you. As a result of your interest and experience, you may undertake the graduate work required to become a fully qualified researcher. It is very important that a number of nurses obtain this type of preparation if nursing is to have the research leadership it needs. As of 1973, the American Nurses' Foundation reported that approximately one thousand nurses in the United States have earned a doctoral degree, the degree that prepares one to do independent research (American Nurses' Foundation, 1973). This number represents approximately one-tenth of one percent of the nursing profession. At least ten times as many nurse researchers are needed.

But suppose you do not wish to be actively involved in research, or do not have an opportunity to be involved. What then? You still have an important responsibility—one that in the long run justifies research. This is the responsibility of making use of findings of scientific inquiry.

As a nurse, whatever your position or wherever you work, you need to keep abreast of the research reported in the literature of your field of interest and to evaluate it. When you find a study that appears to have been soundly done and the conclusions seem logical, you will want to try out the findings in your practice. As you do this you may even find additional areas needing study.

RESEARCH AND NURSING RESEARCH DEFINED

According to *Webster's Seventh New Collegiate Dictionary* (1971), research is a careful or diligent search or "studious inquiry or examination, especially investigations or experimentation aimed at the discovery and interpretation of facts, or practical application of such new or revised theories."

In the strictest sense, nursing research is concerned with the systematic investigation of nursing practice itself, and of the effect of this practice on patient care or on individual, family, or community health. This statement is not meant to imply that research in nursing education or in the administration of nursing service is not vitally important; it is, but it is not strictly nursing research. Rather, it is educational research in nursing, or it is nursing administration research. These approaches are commonly included in the general term nursing research. In fact, all research that is related to nursing, both basic and applied, is considered nursing research by many. Others believe, however, that the term refers to research in nursing practice and in the nursing care needs of patients, that is, clinical research.

SCIENTIFIC INVESTIGATION AND PROBLEM SOLVING

Scientific inquiry is sometimes compared to problem solving, although the latter is simpler than research. Perhaps the best way of comparing the two approaches is to compare their uses.

Problem solving usually involves finding a solution for an immediate, practical problem. That is, it concerns a problem in patient care which cannot wait for research, and consists of the following steps:

1. Becoming aware of the particular problem or condition of the patient or family that requires care.

2. Analyzing the various aspects of the problem; for example, the need for immediate care, the type of care needed, the need to refer the family for social or financial assistance, and the resources available.

3. Collecting data about the patient or family, the problem, and possible solutions through the use of records, observation, interviews, discussion with other professionals familiar with the patient, and review of the pertinent literature.

4. Analyzing the information collected and using this analysis as a guide to action in helping the patient with his problem.

5. Checking with the patient and/or the family to evaluate the effect of the action taken. If the action fails to solve the problem, start over, looking for alternate solutions.

The purpose of research is to provide new knowledge by finding valid answers to questions that have been raised or valid solutions to problems that have been identified. Unlike problem solving, the problem selected for research is not related to a particular patient or immediate concern; rather, it is related to the care of patients generally, or to a particular group of patients, and the expectation is that the results of the research will benefit many patients.

An investigation that seeks to find solutions to a practical problem such as, for example, a problem in clinical nursing practice, is called *applied research*. New knowledge derived from applied research will be useful and can be applied in the field without much delay. *Basic research*, on the other hand, is not concerned with a here-and-now practical problem; it is concerned with the establishment of new knowledge or facts and the development of fundamental theories which will not always be immediately applicable.

Most of the studies in nursing have been applied research. However, both types of research are important and necessary, and more nurses should become interested in basic research. Examples of basic research done by nurses are Kolthoff's study of microcirculation in the skin (1972) and Parson's study "The Effect of Stimulation of the 'Nonspecific Region of the Thalamus' upon the Intracellular Activity of Neurons in the Motor Cortex Made Epileptic with Strychnine" (1972). These two nurses are also physiologists. Their investigations will not produce immediate answers to nursing problems. The knowledge they discover regarding microcirculation in the skin and the basic mechanisms in epilepsy should eventually make a significant contribution to both nursing and physiology by providing basic scientific knowledge upon which further research can be based.

Simply stated, scientific research, basic and applied, involves the following steps:

1. Identifying the problem, delineating it clearly, and delimiting it to a manageable research question or hypothesis (see chapter 3).

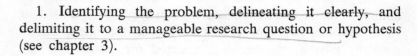

2. Collecting essential facts pertaining to the problem. This includes reviewing the literature, validating the significance of the problem, and selecting or developing theories pertinent to explaining the problem and its possible solution.

3. Developing a tentative solution (or solutions), called a *hypothesis* (or in the plural, hypotheses).

4. Setting up a suitable design or method for the study.

5. Collecting the essential data (facts) required for evaluating the hypothesis.

6. Analyzing and evaluating the data in terms of the hypothesis.

7. Reporting the research and its findings.

Each of the seven steps may be simple or complex, depending on the nature and complexity of the problem studied. Regardless of complexity, however, research must follow these general steps as carefully as possible and be conducted with complete objectivity and honesty.

The implication, then, is that research may be done for one or more of several reasons: (1) to study the various aspects of a problem of care—for example, the exploratory study of the care of patients with indwelling intravenous catheters mentioned earlier (Ross, 1972); (2) to compare two or more methods of care—for example, the structured interview versus the nonstructured one (see Marshall and Feeney, 1972); (3) to evaluate the use of a specific approach to care, which usually involves comparing the approach to one group to that of a control group; or (4) to evaluate a theory of nursing.

To summarize, research may seek new facts by: (1) describing and analyzing a situation or problem; (2) making a critical interpretation of facts already known; or (3) discovering new relationships among facts by means of experimentation. The first type of research commonly involves a descriptive or analytical approach; the second involves a historical or documentary approach; and the third involves an experimental or explanatory approach.

TYPES OF RESEARCH

Descriptive Research

Descriptive research describes what is and analyzes the findings in relation to their significance. Most nursing research is of this type. It is often done for the important purpose of generating hypotheses for future experimental studies, or it may simply be a way of finding out what the facts are (for example, by means of a survey). In nursing there is great need for research that is conducted for the purpose of developing theories or hypotheses to be tested, since "hunches" about approaches to care frequently occur as a result of carefully made and analyzed observations. Collection of such data is, therefore, an important step that frequently needs to be taken prior to the initiation of scientific experimentation. Many different data collection techniques are used in this type of research, including interviewing, making surveys and observations, and preparing case studies. Examples of descriptive research in nursing can readily be found in the literature:

- "I Came, I Saw, I Responded: Nursing Observation and Action Survey," by Verhonick et al. (1968) reported a study of nurses attending two national conventions. Filmed sequences of patient situations were utilized. The purpose of the study was to examine the types of responses that professional nurses would give to the situations observed. The investigators found that the number of relevant observations increased progressively as the level of the academic degree held by the nurse increased.

• A study of the sleep and rest patterns of patients following heart surgery (Walker, 1972) utilized careful clinical observations and their interpretation in terms of their significance for nursing. Despite the limitations of the study (small sample and limited number of observations made), it resulted in a number of hypotheses on which future studies might be based.

• "The Use of Electrocardiograph Monitoring in Nursing Research" (Mansfield, 1966) reported on the use of electrocardiographic monitoring to study the effects of certain activities on the heart action of healthy subjects and those who had had open heart surgery. The investigators noted how various physical activities, interactions, and nursing care activities affected the subjects' electrocardiograms.

• "Behavioral Characteristics of Heroin Addicts on a Short-term Detoxification Program" by Brink (1972) illustrated the use of a descriptive study to delineate the behavior of a specific type of patient and thus added to our knowledge regarding this type of patient.

• In "A Study of Factors Contributing to Skin Breakdown" (Williams, 1972), data on nonambulatory patients were obtained through ratings given to the study subjects' skin condition. Williams correlated the ratings with a number of patient variables and found that body weight and infection (other than genitourinary) had the highest correlation with decubitus formation; that is to say, thin patients with infections were most apt to develop decubitus ulcers.

Historical Research

Historical or *documentary research* is the type least frequently utilized by nurse researchers. There have been few historiographers in our profession, although histories of nursing were compiled by Nutting and Dock (1907), Dock (1912), Dock and Stewart (1920), Stewart and Austin (1962), and others. According to Christy (1972), historical research follows a specific research methodology and is as concerned with validity and reliability of data as are other types of research. This nurse historian has written several carefully researched and documented biographic articles on such leaders in nursing as Annie W. Goodrich, M. Adelaide Nutting, and Lillian Wald (Christy, 1970 a and b; 1969, a, b, c, d).

The Woolsey Sisters by Austin (1971) and Woodham-Smith's *Florence Nightingale* (1951) are examples of carefully documented, book-length biographies. Stella Goostray's *Memoirs: Half a Century in Nursing* is a book of remembrances of one individual and thus may not be as well documented as are biographies; however, such writings are most useful in giving impressions of a period in nursing.

The value of historical research is not merely that it provides a record of the past, but that it contributes to present thought and decision making. The old saying that "history repeats itself" is often interpreted to mean that we tend to repeat our failures. But much can be learned from history that will help to explain the present and to broaden our perspective concerning today's problems. According to one author (Fischer, 1970, pp. 315-316), history's value lies in its ability to help clarify the context in which today's problems exist. Further, it contributes to the solution of future problems by adding another dimension to our theoretical knowledge. (For example, what were the conditions under which nursing made significant progress and those under which it faltered?) It helps to *think* historically, to take stock, and to determine new directions.

For a further exposition of the methods used in historical research, read Christy's (1972) "Characteristics of Historical Research and Problems of the Historian," and Monteiro's "Research into Things Past: Tracking Down One of Miss Nightingale's Correspondents" (1972).

The major techniques used in historical research are documentation of the evidence and evaluation of its authenticity. These techniques stress the use of primary rather than secondary sources and involve both external and internal appraisal. In external appraisal the investigator asks "How genuine is the material?" and "Is it what it purports to be?" In internal appraisal he asks "How trustworthy is the material contained in the document?" Just as in descriptive research, historical research may start with a hunch or hypothesis and it may produce hypotheses or generalizations. For example, one may say that the depression of the 1930s was a direct cause of the decline of private duty nursing in this country; that wars have always advanced the understanding of the need for nursing care; that the status and roles of women have had an influence on the advancement of nursing; and so forth. The increasing number of doctoral dissertations that are based on historical research reflects a growing interest among nurses in this type of research.

Experimental Research

Whereas the investigator who uses the descriptive method makes his observations under natural conditions, one using the *experimental* or *explanatory* method manipulates the situation in some way in order to test the hypothesis, or hypotheses, that have been made. A controlled situation is set up; that is, certain factors, or variables, are held constant and an independent or experimental variable is manipulated and the results evaluated and compared with the results obtained in the controlled group (see chapter 6 for definitions of these terms). Usually at least one control and one experimental group are used.

The purposes of experimental studies may be to determine or explain why something happens, to see whether a predicted result occurs when a specific type of care is given, or to evaluate a new program or project. The continuing development of nursing science is in no small part dependent upon sound experimental research. Some examples of this type of research in nursing include:

• "Nursing Intervention with the Presurgical Patient: Effectiveness and Efficiency of Group and Individual Preoperative Teaching—Phase Two," by Lindeman (1972). In this study the investigator compared the effect of individual teaching with that of group teaching on length of learning time, on postoperative need for analgesics, on postoperative ventilatory functioning, and on length of hospitalization. She found group teaching to be just as effective as and more efficient than individual patient teaching.

• "The Impact of Physical-Physiological Activity on Infants' Growth and Development," by Porter (1972). This study compared the growth and development of infants who received cycling motion exercises over a two-month period with the growth and development of a control group who did not receive these exercises. The greater increase in growth and development of the infants in the experimental group supported the hypothesis on which the research was based.

• "Auditory Stimulation and Developmental Behavior in the Premature Infant," by Katz (1971). Thirty-one experimental and 31 control infants were studied to test the hypothesis that those subjected to a regimen of maternal auditory stimulation would show significantly greater maturational development. The findings supported the hypothesis and the investigator suggests that in our zeal to protect the premature infant from infection we may be creating a sensory deficit.

ETHICAL ASPECTS OF NURSING RESEARCH

In recent years considerable concern has been expressed about the protection of the rights of individuals used as subjects of research. Factors involved in such protection are: (1) informed consent on the part of the subject, (2) confidentiality of the data collected, and (3) protection of the individual from harm.

In 1968 the Board of Directors of the American Nurses' Association approved a statement entitled "Guidelines on Ethical Values," which outlined the responsibilities of the researcher in protecting human rights (American Nurses' Association, 1968). The guidelines include discussions of: (1) the right to privacy (anonymity and the amount the subject will divulge), (2) the right of self-determination (informed consent), (3) the right of conservation of personal resources (time, energy, etc.), (4) the right to freedom from arbitrary hurt (arbitrary physical or mental suffering), (5) the right to freedom from intrinsic risk of injury (emotional or physical), and (6) the rights of minors or incompetent persons (informed consent of relatives).

Today, most institutions in which research involving humans is carried out have a committee that reviews all research proposals. Their review is concerned not only with the significance of the study and the soundness of the research design but also with the evidence that the subjects' rights will be protected. The committee's review and approval become particularly important when the full nature of the research purpose cannot be disclosed to the subjects.

The factor of informed consent must be given careful consideration. If you plan a research project in which human beings are the subjects, you need to consider the kind of explanation that will be required for the subject to understand the nature of the project. It may not be necessary to give a complete description of the project and its purposes, if doing so would ruin your chances of obtaining the data you need. For example, in the Waters et al. (1972) study of technical and professional nursing, participation in the study was requested of the nurses selected. The nurse subjects were told that they were to be observed and interviewed as part of a study of patient care decision making, but they were not told that professional and technical nursing would be compared, since this knowledge might have colored their actions during the observation and their responses in the interview.

SUMMARY

In this chapter we have discussed why research is done, the responsibility that you as a nurse have for participating in research, and the ethical considerations involved in all research. We have also explained the types of research and given examples of each.

Research is serious business. It should not be entered into lightly, but neither should it be feared. It can be the most exciting, demanding, and rewarding of experiences for the amateur as well as the "pro."

REFERENCES

American Nurses' Association. *The Nurse in Research: ANA Guidelines on Ethical Values.* New York, The Association, January 1968. (Also in *Nurs Res* 17:104–107, Mar.-Apr. 1968.)

American Nurses' Foundation. *International Directory of Nurses with Doctoral Degrees.* New York, The Foundation, 1973.

Austin, Anne L. *The Woolsey Sisters of New York, 1860–1900.* Philadelphia, American Philosophical Society, 1971.

Brink, Pamela J. Behavioral characteristics of heroin addicts on a short-term detoxification program. *Nurs Res* 21:38–45, Jan.-Feb. 1972.

Christy, Teresa E. Characteristics of historical research and problems of the historian. In *American Nurses' Association Eighth Nursing Research Conference,* Albuquerque, New Mexico, March 15–17, 1972. New York, The Association, 1972, pp. 227–228.

———. Portrait of a leader: Lillian D. Wald. *Nurs Outlook* 18:50–54, Mar. 1970 (a).

———. Portrait of a leader: Annie Warburton Goodrich. *Nurs Outlook* 18:46–50, Aug. 1970 (b).

———. Portrait of a leader: M. Adelaide Nutting. *Nurs Outlook* 17:20–24, Jan. 1969 (a).

———. Portrait of a leader: Isabel Hampton Robb. *Nurs Outlook* 17:26–29, Mar. 1969 (b).

———. Portrait of a leader: Lavinia Lloyd Dock. *Nurs Outlook* 17:72–75, June 1969 (c).

———. Portrait of a leader: Isabel Maitland Stewart. *Nurs Outlook* 17:44–48, Oct. 1969 (d).

Cornell, Sudie A. et al. Comparison of three bowel management programs during rehabilitation of spinal cord injured patients. *Nurs Res* 22:321–328, July-Aug. 1973.

Dock, Lavinia L. *A History of Nursing.* Vols. 3 and 4. New York, Putnam, 1912.

Dock, Lavinia L. and Stewart, Isabel M. *A Short History of Nursing.* New York, Putnam, 1920.

Fischer, David H. *Historians' Fallacies: Toward a Logic of Historical Thought.* New York, Harper and Row, 1970.

Goostray, Stella. *Memoirs: Half a Century in Nursing.* Boston, Nursing Archive, Mugar Memorial Library, Boston University, 1969.

Katz, Violet. Auditory stimulation and developmental behavior in the premature infant. *Nurs Res* 20:196–201, May-June 1971.

Kolthoff, Norma J. Microcirculation in human skin. In *American Nurses' Association Eighth Nursing Research Conference,* Albuquerque, New Mexico, March 15–17, 1972. New York, The Association, 1972, pp. 87–100.

Lindeman, Carol A. Nursing intervention with the presurgical patient: effectiveness and efficiency of group and individual preoperative teaching—phase II. *Nurs Res* 21:196–209, May-June 1972.

Mansfield, Louise W. The use of electrocardiographic monitoring in nursing research. In *American Nurses' Association Second Nursing Research Conference,* Phoenix, Arizona, February 28, March 1–2, 1966. New York, The Association, 1966, pp. 100–137.

Marshall, Jon C. and Feeney, Sally. Structured versus intuitive intake interview. *Nurs Res* 21:269–272, July-Aug. 1972.

Monteiro, Lois. Research into things past: tracking down one of Miss Nightingale's correspondents. *Nurs Res* 21:526–529, Nov.-Dec. 1972.

Nutting, Mary A. and Dock, Lavinia L. *A History of Nursing.* Vols. 1 and 2. New York, Putnam, 1907.

Parsons, L. Claire. The effect of stimulation of the "nonspecific region of the thalamus" upon the intracellular activity of neurons in the motor cortex made epileptic with strychnine. In *American Nurses' Association Eighth Nursing Research Conference,* Albuquerque, New Mexico, March 15–17, 1972. New York, The Association, 1972, pp. 101–112.

Porter, Luz S. The impact of physical-physiological activity on infants' growth and development. *Nurs Res* 21:210–219, May-June 1972.

Ross, S. Ann. Infusion phlebitis: selected factors. *Nurs Res* 21: 313–318, July-Aug. 1972.

Stewart, Isabel M. and Austin, Anne L. *A History of Nursing.* New York, Putnam, 1962.

Verhonick, Phyllis J.; Nichols, Glennadee A.; Glor, Beverly A. K.; and McCarthy, Rosemary T. I came, I saw, I responded: nursing observation and action survey. *Nurs Res* 17:38–44, Jan.-Feb. 1968.

Walker, Betty Boyd. The postsurgery heart patient: amount of uninterrupted time for sleep and rest during the first, second, and third postoperative days in a teaching hospital. *Nurs Res* 21:164–169, Mar.-Apr. 1972.

Waters, Verle H.; Chater, Shirley S.; Vivier, Mary L.; Urrea, Judithe H.; and Wilson, Holly S. Technical and professional nursing: an exploratory study. *Nurs Res* 21:124–131, Mar.-Apr. 1972.

Williams, Anne. A study of factors contributing to skin breakdown. *Nurs Res* 21:238–243, May-June 1972.

Woodham-Smith, Cecil. *Florence Nightingale.* New York, McGraw-Hill, 1951.

II

THE RESEARCH PROCESS

3

SELECTING A PROBLEM

As we have found in the two preceding chapters, the purpose of research is to discover unknown facts, explanations, interpretations, and relationships among facts. We have also learned that research may be either basic or applied, descriptive, experimental, or historical. From now on, we shall focus on research in clinical nursing, that is, on studies of nursing practice or of the effect of nursing practice on patient care or on individual, family, or community health situations. Our purpose will be to find out how we can systematically discover facts or identify relationships among facts which will help us solve problems in nursing.

The problems investigated in nursing may be relatively simple ones, or they may be so broad and complex as to involve large groups of nurses or patients and thus require a team approach. An example of a simple problem might be the one studied by Brink (1972)—"Behavioral Characteristics of Heroin Addicts on a Short-Term Detoxification Program"—in which 42 heroin addicts in one institution were studied over a five-month period. An example of the more complex problem might be the one studied by Georgopoulos and Jackson (1970)—"Nursing Kardex Behavior in an Experimental Study of Patient Units with and without Clinical Nurse Specialists." This latter investigation was part of a larger study and involved six 25-bed units, three experimental units led by clinical nurse specialists, and three control units led by conventional head nurses. Individual Kardexes of 764 patients were analyzed. As you can easily see, a study of this kind would require a team of researchers from various fields and a variety of resources. On the other hand, a team may consist of nurses only, which was the approach in the Cornell et al. (1973) study mentioned in chapter 2. These nurses identified the problem and set up the study. Imagine the excitement of designing your own research, reporting the results, and basing your own nursing care on the findings!

FINDING A PROBLEM

How does one go about choosing a problem to study? You may already have in mind a suitable question about some aspect of patient care which has grown out of your daily work or your background of experiences. For instance, you may have been questioning, as McBride (1967) did, whether nurses' approaches to patients might have an effect on the relief of their pain. On the other hand, you may not have any questions or hunches about ways of improving care but are interested in doing some research. In that case, you might go to the literature and read some of the studies reported in the various nursing journals. This will give you a picture of the many kinds of problems other nurses have observed, and such an excursion may stimulate your imagination so that you will soon discover that you have several questions of your own that fall into the "What is ————?" or the "Why is such and such happening?" category. This is the beginning of the intellectual curiosity that is so essential to problem identification.

Of course, the literature is also full of suggestions for study. Many investigations raise as many, if not more, questions than they answer. You might even decide to replicate a reported study in order to substantiate, or perhaps refute, its findings.

A good review of the literature in your particular area of interest is not only an excellent source of problems but will also serve to enrich your background and help you to relate your interests to those of others in the same field. This is not the same kind of review of the literature that you will do after you have selected your problem. You need to have as much understanding of the general area as you can get before deciding upon a particular problem. Perhaps you have specialized in the area of your subject and do not need this review, but, even if you are familiar with the literature, a review will refresh your knowledge of the area.

Suppose the question you are interested in relates to the use of programmed instruction in teaching diabetic patients. You would need to be thoroughly familiar not only with the subject of diabetes and the care of diabetic patients but also with the subject of health teaching methods, including programmed instruction. If you had not already acquired this familiarity, now would be the time to do so.

DELIMITING THE PROBLEM

Some problems, of course, may not be researchable. They may be so global that they do not lend themselves to study. A question such as "How can I improve the self-care of diabetic patients?" would be much too broad, although it could well be the first question you ask. "What is the most effective method of teaching diabetic patients how to take their own insulin?" would also be rather indefinite, although, again, you might start with this question. (Time for teaching is often difficult to find in a busy clinic and, in addition, you want to find the most successful way of teaching patients.) A much more specific question would be "Can diabetic patients learn to care for themselves and to take their own insulin as effectively through the use of programmed instruction as by means of group instruction?" This question could be studied by making a systematic comparison of the two teaching methods.

The next step in determining whether a problem is researchable, or at least whether you would be able to study it, is to determine whether the appropriate patients and the resources needed to do the study are available to you. For example, if you are teaching diabetic patients, it might be relatively easy for you to plan a comparative study of the two methods of teaching suggested earlier if resources for making use of the two methods are available. You may have been using the group method of teaching. However, at a nurses' meeting you heard about a programmed instruction booklet which would appear to offer a more effective method, and you want to try it. Is the booklet available for your use? If not, would it be possible to find another? Or, would it be possible for you to develop one yourself? The answers to these questions would help you decide on the practicality of the problem for study, but you would also need to know if methods of comparing the results are available. You might decide to pre- and posttest your patients in some way and to develop the tests yourself, perhaps with the help of experts. Also, expert opinion might be available for helping you develop a rating scale for evaluating such variables as skin condition, number of complications, handling of injections, and urine testing, to mention a few. You probably would also want to find out about additional ways of rating the effectiveness or outcomes of the two teaching methods.

You may think that we have made much ado about selecting a problem for study. However, this is one of the most important steps in the whole research process and determines to a large extent the nature and quality of your research. It is often said that once we know what the problem is, we are well on our way to solving it.

Problem identification is not always easy. However, the habit of systematic observation plus intellectual curiosity and a questioning attitude will help. A further help is familiarity with the literature, which will provide suggestions for problems that need to be studied.

ESTABLISHING THE SIGNIFICANCE OF THE PROBLEM

An important factor in the selection of a problem for study is whether it is an important or significant one. Is there a real need to find an answer to it? As you review the literature, particularly the research literature, you will see that in most reports the introductory material provides a rationale for the study; that is, it explains the reason why the investigator considered the study to be important. On the face of it, the suggested study of the use of programmed instruction would appear to be of importance in that improved learning by diabetic patients should result in better self-care and fewer complications. However, if several scientific investigations of this problem, using programmed instruction to advantage, have already been reported in the literature, you might question the need for doing another one. Nevertheless, the study would be in order if some new element has been added to the instruction method since these studies were made, or if your evaluation of the studies suggests a need for substantiating the findings.

STATING THE PURPOSE

Once you have identified the problem, you can come up with a clear statement of your purpose in studying it. This will give direction and focus to the study. For example, the purpose of the study we suggested would be to compare the effectiveness of two methods of teaching diabetic patients self-care—group instruction and programmed instruction. The purpose of the Brink study (1972) mentioned earlier was to determine characteristic patterns of behavior in heroin addicts on a short-term detoxification program. One may argue that the purpose of both studies would be to improve the care of certain patients. This is the ultimate purpose of all nursing research and an indication of the usefulness of the particular study. Although some researchers do include the ultimate reason for the study (to plan better care for these patients, for example), this is not necessarily part of the specific statement of purpose.

The rationale for a study often includes not only the statement of the problem but also the significance and usefulness of the study. The rationale should clearly tie in with and culminate in the statement of the purpose of the research. In the suggested study of methods of teaching the diabetic patient, for example, the importance of teaching these patients effectively would have to be established. Next would come the determination of the need for a solution of the question about the use of programmed instruction. These two steps would logically lead to a statement of the purpose of the study.

SUMMARY

Selecting a problem, determining its significance or importance, and relating these factors to one's understanding of the purpose of nursing research are all necessary before starting a research project. It is important to remember that the statement of the problem to be studied and the statement of the purpose of the study are not the same. The problem is a question that needs to be answered, or an unsatisfactory condition for which a solution is sought; the purpose is the aim of the study, which may be to describe, to explain, or to predict something related to the problem's solution.

REFERENCES

Brink, Pamela J. Behavioral characteristics of heroin addicts on a short-term detoxification program. *Nurs Res* 21:38–45, Jan.-Feb. 1972.

Cornell, Sudie A. et al. Comparison of three bowel management programs during rehabilitation of spinal cord injured patients. *Nurs Res* 22:321–328, July-Aug. 1973.

Georgopoulos, Basil S. and Jackson, Marjorie M. Nursing Kardex behavior in an experimental study of patient units with and without clinical nurse specialists. *Nurs Res* 19:196–218, May-June 1970.

McBride, Mary Angela B. Nursing approach, pain and relief: an exploratory experiment. *Nurs Res* 16:337–341, Fall 1967.

4

THE LITERATURE SEARCH

After you have decided on the problem you want to study, you will need to do a bit of reading to find out what has already been researched in the area and to get all the ideas you can to help you develop your hypothesis and decide on the research methods you will use. The first search of the literature helps one to identify and select a research problem, but the second search should be confined to investigating materials that are directly relevant to the problem to be solved.

A careful, systematic literature review will include recent publications and will go back as far as is consistent with the nature of the problem chosen for study. It must be sufficiently thorough to familiarize the researcher with past studies that are pertinent to the one now being planned. For example, if one is interested in studying the effect of various preoperative nursing approaches on the postoperative recovery of the patient who is facing a mutilative type of surgery, one may need to search the literature for studies of the effect of nursing approaches, studies based upon interpersonal interaction, studies of the effect of mutilating surgery, and studies of the effect of specific types of preoperative care on postoperative recovery. Each such study may suggest additional studies that should be examined.

DOCUMENTING THE SEARCH

Every study reviewed in a literature search should be evaluated as to its strengths and limitations, methods used, results obtained, and relevance to the study being planned. A file should be kept on all references reviewed and each entry should include the complete citation of the reference; that is, author(s) name(s); title of the report, article, or book; name of journal or publisher; date of publication; pages on which the material appears; and the notes you have made on it. Careful note-taking and reference citation will save many headaches later when you get into the study and when you prepare the report.

LOCATING THE RELEVANT LITERATURE

The most important resource for a literature search is a good library. Every nurse should develop skill in the use of this resource. If you need assistance in learning how to make the best use of the library, the librarian can be most helpful in explaining the use of catalog cards, indexes, abstracts, and directories, as well as a wealth of other tools, all designed to open doors to the available literature.

Nursing is very fortunate in having a number of important tools that give access to the nursing literature. Abstracts of studies in nursing have appeared in the journal *Nursing Research* since 1959. They cover studies in public health nursing from 1924 on, and other studies in nursing or relevant to nursing from 1955 on. Henderson's *Nursing Studies Index,* a four-volume annotated index, lists all studies reported during the period from 1900 to 1959. Other indexes include the *Cumulative Index to Nursing Literature,* which covers the period from 1956 on, the *International Nursing Index (INI)*, which lists worldwide nursing literature from 1966 on, and, of course, the annual indexes to the various nursing periodicals.

The nurse researcher may also want to make use of related reference tools in the fields of medicine, biology, sociology, psychology, or education. Guides to the various types of tools are available. See, for example, "Reference Tools for Nurses" in Spalding and Notter (1970); Parkin's (1972) "Information Resources for Nursing Research"; and "Reference Sources for Nursing" in the May 1972 issue of *Nursing Outlook.* Information about resources in fields other than nursing may be in one of the guides to library use such as Gate's (1969) *Guide to the Use of Books and Libraries* and *The New York Times Guide to Reference Materials* (McCormick, 1971).

Today, nursing has an additional access service known as MEDLINE which the National Library of Medicine makes available through its regional library centers, medical schools, and hospital and medical or health science libraries. This service, instituted in 1972, provides telephone access to a number of medical and health-related journals. It can furnish immediate access to citations to literature that has been identified but has not had time to appear in the *INI* or in *Index Medicus.* Thirteen leading nursing journals currently indexed in *INI* are included in MEDLINE, and it is hoped that more will be added as the service continues.

PRIMARY AND SECONDARY SOURCES

When doing a literature search one must be careful to differentiate between *primary* and *secondary* sources. A reference to a piece of research by someone other than the original researcher is not the same thing as a reference to a report by the person who did the study. Also, while abstracts of studies are important as a way of locating relevant studies, they should not be cited as references because information contained in abstracts or other secondary sources is summarized and may include interpretations by the abstractor, or even inaccuracies. To be sure of the facts and to be able to draw your own conclusions, you need to read the original, or primary, source.

Differentiation between primary and secondary sources is of vital importance in historical research in which one must examine the actual records rather than accounts of what is in the records. It is equally important in the literature search in descriptive and experimental studies, each of which has its documentation stage, i.e., the literature review.

RELATIONSHIP OF SEARCH TO RATIONALE

The importance of identifying the significance of your study for nursing was mentioned in the foregoing chapter. The literature search should contribute to your argument for the importance of the investigation. Information gleaned from the literature should help you to delineate the boundaries of the problem more clearly, to discuss it in relation to previous studies and show how it differs from others, and to indicate how this study is expected to add to our knowledge and improve our practice.

The search may also unearth theories related to the solution of your problem. Therefore, it is important to be on the lookout for theories which offer promising explanations for the phemonenon under study.

SUMMARY

The literature review required before undertaking a research project is somewhat like the work of a detective, and it can be equally fascinating. Each new find becomes more exciting than the last, especially if it brings new understanding of the problem or an idea for the research method that might be employed.

While the researcher tries to limit her reading to relevant topics, she also may have the experience of getting off the main path and being lured into interesting bypaths. If you suddenly find yourself reading something that has captured your interest but which has absolutely nothing to do with your study, do not be surprised. This is not an uncommon experience. It may even lead to the development of other problems you will want to study later. However, such detours should be kept to a minimum, and self-discipline may be needed at times to keep your focus on your main concern—the literature that is relevant to your current study.

If your reading is well directed, you will come up with a carefully thought-out problem that is related to the research in the area and, if pertinent, with a theory that can be tested by your study. If your work is well done, you will be ready for the next step, the development of a hypothesis to be tested.

REFERENCES

Abstracts of Studies in Nursing 1955–1958. *Nurs Res* 9:51–117, Spring 1960. (Abstracts have appeared in every issue of *Nursing Research* from 1960 to the present.)

Abstracts of Studies in Public Health Nursing 1924–1957. *Nurs Res* 8:45–115, Spring 1959.

Committee of the Interagency Council on Library Resources for Nursing. References sources for nursing. *Nurs Outlook* 20:338–343, May 1972.

Cumulative Index to Nursing Literature. Glendale, California, Glendale Adventist Hospital, 1956 to present.

Gates, Jean K. *Guide to the Use of Books and Libraries.* 2nd ed. New York, McGraw-Hill, 1969.

Henderson, Virginia, et al. *Nursing Studies Index.* Vols. 1–4, 1900–1959. Philadelphia, J. B. Lippincott, Vol. 1, 1972; Vol. 2, 1970; Vol. 3, 1966; Vol. 4, 1963. (Vol. 1 covers the period 1900 to 1929; Vol. 2, the period 1930 to 1949; Vol. 3, the period 1950 to 1956; Vol. 4, the period 1957 to 1959.)

International Nursing Index. New York, The American Journal of Nursing Company, 1966 to present.

McCormick, Mona. *The New York Times Guide to Reference Materials.* New York, Popular Library, 1971 (paperback). (Original title: *Who-What-When-Where-How-Why-Made Easy)*

Parkin, Margaret L. Information resources for nursing research. *Canadian Nurse* 68:40–43, Mar. 1972.

Spalding, Eugenia K. and Notter, Lucille E. *Professional Nursing: Foundations, Perspectives, and Relationships.* 8th ed. Philadelphia, J. B. Lippincott Co., 1970. See Appendix, Part 1, Reference Materials for Nurses, pp. 639–648.

5

THE HYPOTHESIS

A statement of the predicted relationships between the factors one wishes to analyze, i.e., the *variables* in a study, is known as the *hypothesis*. The hypothesis grows out of the problem to be studied and the theoretical framework that has been developed for the study. It is a tentative solution or explanation of the problem which the investigator has arrived at through his review of the literature—in other words, a theory that he has found which appears to explain the situation or one he has developed on the basis of his own experience.

Thus, it is apparent that hypotheses are not just guesses. They may be based on hunches in the beginning, but by the time the study actually gets under way these hunches have been refined into a carefully thought-out statement of the problem and are supported by a rationale based upon a review of the relevant literature.

PURPOSE OF THE HYPOTHESIS

That formulating the hypothesis is a very important step in any research project becomes evident when we consider that the hypothesis determines the type of study that will be done and the variables that will be studied. An examination of the following three hypotheses, proposed by Lindeman and Van

Aernam (1971) in their study of the effect of nursing intervention on the care of the presurgical patient, will show this relationship:

1. Structured preoperative teaching would significantly increase the adult surgical patient's ability to cough and deep breathe as measured by his vital capacity, maximum expiratory flow rate, and forced expiratory volume.
2. Structured preoperative teaching would significantly reduce [the] average length of hospital stay for the adult surgical patient.
3. Structured preoperative teaching would significantly reduce the need for postoperative analgesics for the adult surgical patient (p. 321).

Obviously, these hypotheses identify: (1) the population that will be studied—adult surgical patients; (2) the problem solution that has been selected—structured preoperative teaching; (3) the variables to be studied—coughing and deep breathing, length of hospital stay, need for postoperative analgesics, and structured teaching versus nonstructured teaching; and (4) measurements to be used—vital capacity, maximum expiratory flow rate, forced expiratory volume, length of hospitalization, and number of analgesics prescribed. These hypotheses also provide for an experimental design, that is, an experimental group would receive the structured teaching and a control group would receive nonstructured teaching.

It should be noted that these hypotheses flowed directly from the description of the problem (the continued occurrence of postoperative respiratory and circulatory complications) and from the presence of many unanswered questions about the stir-up routine and about teaching this routine to patients.

In this study, the hypotheses predicted the results the experimenters expected to obtain. Such a prediction does not indicate a bias on the part of the investigator; it simply provides a framework for the study. The design of the study must preserve the objectivity of the experiment, and the results will permit either acceptance or nonacceptance of the hypotheses.

Some investigators use what is known as the *null hypothesis*. Instead of predicting a significant relationship between the independent variable and the dependent variables, (see chapter 6), they predict no significant relationship. The null hypothesis is related to the statistical test to be used (see chapter 8). Rejection of the null hypothesis indicates that there is a significant difference between the groups examined.

THEORETICAL FRAMEWORK AND THE HYPOTHESIS

Not only does the nature of the problem influence the hypothesis, but the *theoretical framework* of the study is also directly related to it. In the Lindeman-Van Aernam (1971) study, no theoretical framework was reported; had there been, it would have been reflected in the hypotheses. A recent study that did use a theoretical framework was reported by Porter (1972). Her study of the effect of physical activity (passive cycling exercises) on infants' growth and development was based on two theories: that growth and development are unitary and integrative and that the human organism is an open system which interacts constantly with the environment. The researcher's hypothesis reflected this theoretical framework in that it embodied the idea that infants who received physical and emotional support plus passive cycling exercises (planned physical-physiological activity) would show greater increases in growth and development on specific indexes (weight, length, motor behavior, language behavior, adaptive behavior, and personal/social behavior) than would infants who received only physical care and emotional support.

Thus, the use of theory can be an important technique in developing a conceptual framework for a study, and this conceptual framework will, in turn, influence the nature of the hypothesis.

IS A HYPOTHESIS ALWAYS NECESSARY?

Although formulating the hypothesis is a necessary step in explanatory or experimental research, it may or may not be required in descriptive research. Some descriptive studies are exploratory in nature and may actually be done in order to generate hypotheses. The Brink (1972) study was of this nature. Its purpose was simply to identify and document characteristic behavior patterns of heroin addicts on a short-term detoxification program. The findings contribute to our knowledge of the behavior of such patients and can be used in planning nursing care or in the development of hypotheses for future studies.

Other studies are conducted for the purpose of raising questions for future investigation, either because not enough is known about the problem or because the investigator is not yet ready to develop specific hypotheses. Davitz and Pendleton (1969) illustrate this approach in their studies of nurses' inferences about pain others feel. They raised four questions as bases for four studies:

> Do nurses from different cultural and subcultural groups infer varying degrees of suffering in response to identical stimuli? (p. 101)

> Does the degree of inferred suffering in patients vary as a function of the clinical specialty of the nurse? (p. 103)

What are the varying degrees of suffering nurses associate with a diagnosis of depression, leukemia, diabetes, and second- and third-degree burns? (p. 104)

Do age, sex, and socioeconomic class of the patient influence the nurse's inference of the degree of suffering? (p. 105)

All four of these studies resulted in identifying important specific areas for future study, three of which have been carried out and reported in the literature under the overall title "Inferences of Physical Pain and Psychological Distress" (Baer, Davitz, and Lieb, 1970; Lenburg, Glass, and Davitz, 1970; Lenburg, Burnside, and Davitz, 1970).

Another type of investigation that does not require the statement of a hypothesis is one that is done primarily to test a research instrument. Such a study is necessary when there are no known tested instruments that can be used for investigating a particular problem, since use of an untested instrument may well create lack of confidence in the study findings. Graffam's (1970) study "Nurse Response to the Patient in Distress—Development of an Instrument" is an example of instrument testing. The investigator documented the need for an instrument to use in her study of nurses' responses to patients' complaints of distress; she described the development of the instrument to be used in observing the nurse—a checklist that included demographic data on the patient (age, sex, race, diagnosis); day, date, and timing of the event recorded; and, finally, data about the complaint and the nurse's response to it.

After the instrument being tested has met the criteria of validity and reliability, the investigator can move on to the next stage of the research, the testing of her hypotheses. In this case, the hypotheses were that registering of complaints by patients is a complex process and that nurses often make automatic, impersonal, and limited responses to these complaints.

SUMMARY

We have given considerable attention to the hypothesis because of its great importance in an investigator's preparation for a study. The following chapter, which deals with research method, will bring out the close relationship of the hypothesis to the research method used.

REFERENCES

Baer, Eva; Davitz, Lois J.; and Lieb, Renee. Inferences of physical pain and psychological distress. I. In relation to verbal and nonverbal patient communication. *Nurs Res* 19:388–392, Sept.-Oct. 1970.

Brink, Pamela J. Behavioral characteristics of heroin addicts on a short-term detoxification program. *Nurs Res* 21:38–45, Jan.-Feb. 1972.

Davitz, Lois J. and Pendleton, Sidney H. Nurses' inferences of suffering. *Nurs Res* 18:100–107, Mar.-Apr. 1969.

Graffam, Shirley R. Nurse response to the patient in distress—development of an instrument. *Nurs Res* 19:331–336, July-Aug. 1970.

Lenburg, Carrie B.; Burnside, Helen; and Davitz, Lois J. Inferences of physical pain and psychological distress. III. In relation to length of time in the nursing education program. *Nurs Res* 19:399–401, Sept.-Oct. 1970.

Lenburg, Carrie B.; Glass, Helen P.; and Davitz, Lois J. Inferences of physical pain and psychological distress. II. In relation to the stage of the patient's illness and occupation of the perceiver. *Nurs Res* 19:392–398, Sept.-Oct. 1970.

Lindeman, Carol A. and Van Aernam, Betty. Nursing intervention with the presurgical patient—the effects of structured and unstructured preoperative teaching. *Nurs Res* 20:319–332, July-Aug. 1971.

Porter, Luz S. The impact of physical-physiological activity on infants' growth and development. *Nurs Res* 21:210–219, May-June 1972.

6

THE RESEARCH METHOD

Once the researcher has selected the problem she wishes to study, reviewed the literature, and developed the hypothesis, she is ready to begin work on the design for the study. Identifying the type of problem to be solved and stating the purpose of the study will reveal whether it will be a descriptive, experimental, or historical study and thus will dictate the research method she will employ.

For any discussion of research method to be meaningful to the neophyte, certain frequently used terms need to be defined. For example, the terms "independent variable" and "dependent variable" are commonly used in experimental research and may be mentioned in descriptive studies. A *variable* is any factor, characteristic, quality, or attribute under study. An *independent variable* is one that the investigator manipulates or introduces into the situation; it is also sometimes called the *manipulated variable*. A *dependent variable* is one that is under observation by the investigator in order to note the effect on it of the introduction of an independent variable; it is the terminal outcome or behavior and is sometimes called the *criterion variable*. In the Lindeman-Van Aernam (1971) study discussed in chapter 5, the independent or manipulated variable was the teaching method used. The experimenters introduced the variable, structured teaching, in order to compare the results with nonstructured teaching. The dependent variables were ability to cough and to deep breathe, length of hospital stay, and number of postoperative analgesics prescribed.

Often, other variables in an experiment will need to be controlled. These are called *control variables* by some (Hulicka and Hulicka, 1962, p. 101). Unless these variables are controlled or held constant, they intervene and affect the results, making it hard to know whether the independent variable or one of these intervening variables caused the effect found. For example, in the Lindeman–Van Aernam (1971) study, certain controls were established for the selection of subjects in order to hold constant the following variables: age, condition on admission, type of surgery, type of anesthesia, ability to cooperate in the ventilatory function tests, and the fact that the patient was not on intermittent positive pressure breathing therapy. In other situations, the time of day that observations are made may be important or, as would be the case in thermometer studies, temperature of the room and whether the patient is febrile.

You can probably think of a number of other variables that it may be important to control in certain studies. In any event, it is always wise to try to equate the control variables in the experimental and the control groups in order to make sure you are free to concentrate on the independent and dependent variables in the study.

A *criterion measure* is a characteristic quality or attribute that can be used to measure the effect of the independent variable upon the subjects studied. Some of the simple, easy-to-apply criterion measures are temperature, blood pressure, and inches in length. Those that involve quality are more difficult to apply. However, errors can occur in even so simple a task as reading the patient's temperature; studies have shown how inaccurate these readings can be. Hence, careful investigators make every effort to ensure accuracy of measurement. For a report of an investigation of the problems an observer encountered in a study on the measurement of blood pressure, see Wilcox's "Observer Factors in the Measurement of Blood Pressure" (1961).

THE DESCRIPTIVE STUDY DESIGN

The descriptive study is the most common type of study used in nursing research. For example, Williams (1972) said that she planned to identify and describe the characteristics of nonambulatory patients who ultimately develop skin breakdown, and thus suggested in the very beginning that her study would be descriptive. She presented no hypotheses; in essence, her research question was: What are the factors that lead to decubitus ulcer formation?

Williams did make some assumptions, however. She assumed that nonambulatory patients will be more likely to have skin breakdown than those who are ambulatory, that other assessable factors besides pressure may be associated with the formation of decubitus ulcers, and that if the patients in her sample were going to develop decubitus ulcers they would do so within four weeks. Not all researchers state their assumptions this explicitly; sometimes assumptions are simply implied. But stating them helps to define further the method to be used; Williams' sample included bedfast or chairfast patients observed over a period of at least four weeks.

Next, in order to collect the desired data from the patients studied, Williams found she needed to develop an assessment tool. She used the literature, the experience of others, and her own experience to develop a tool which was actually a rating scale. She tested this scale in a small *pilot study* (i.e., a study made to test procedures or tools), made a few changes in it, and decided that two evaluations a week on each patient would be sufficient to furnish the data she needed.

Williams collected her data in such a way that each independent variable (body weight, sex, edema, etc.) could be correlated with the criterion measure (i.e., the dependent variable or measured outcome), decubitus ulcer formation. Thus, a design for a *correlational survey* (one made to collect data from a group on more than one variable in order to estimate the relationship between the variables [Fox, 1970, p. 192]) grew from the investigator's statement of purpose and from the problem in which she was interested.

The Williams study is also an example of a *longitudinal survey* (although it was short in terms of time) rather than a *cross-sectional one*. Although either type of survey may be used to study change over a period of time, the longitudinal survey was both appropriate and feasible for studying such a problem as the formation of decubitus ulcers. Sometimes a longitudinal survey is not feasible because of the time involved, and as a result the sample that is selected cuts across the time periods. For example, if an investigator wished to observe changes in students in a certain program, he might employ a cross-sectional survey and observe students at each level of the program rather than following students in one group through their entire education program and into their graduate experience. A comparative study of nursing students' and graduate nurses' attitudes toward death (Golub and Reznikoff, 1971) furnishes a case in point. The investigators assumed that the use of undergraduate student and graduate nurse groups would result in findings that would, for all practical purposes, be as useful as those that would result from a study which followed the students through their graduate experience. Practical decisions of this kind often need to be made but, when they are, the investigators must take into consideration the possible presence of uncontrolled intervening factors that will influence the outcome.

Surveys may be *comparative* or *evaluative* in nature. A survey that is done to obtain facts about the similarities and dissimilarities between the concept of the need for continuity of care held by nurses working in hospitals and that held by nurses working in community health agencies could be comparative in nature (see Dawson and Stern, 1973). A survey done to obtain data about the differences in characteristics of students from three types of basic nursing education programs could be evaluative (see Richards, 1972).

The *case study*, although not often reported in the nursing literature, is basically an in-depth survey that utilizes one subject. This research method is most frequently used to report studies in psychiatric nursing. An interesting example of the case study method is "Tactile Contact: A Measure of Therapeutic Progress" (Daly and Carr, 1967). These authors presented a summary of a case study, but ordinarily case studies are presented in considerable detail with descriptions of the patient's behavior and of the interactions between nurse and patient, and an interpretation of the meaning of the behavior.

THE EXPERIMENTAL STUDY DESIGN

The "true" experimental design has been described by Campbell and Stanley (1963, p. 8). This design was followed by Porter (1972) in her study "The Impact of Physical-Physiological Activity on Infants' Growth and Development" (see chapter 5). Porter's hypothesis, that gains in growth and development of normal full-term infants would result from planned passive cycling exercises, indicated that her study should be experimental. Further, her hypothesis reflected the criterion measures she would use to determine gains in length and weight and in motor, language, adaptive, and personal/social behaviors. She carefully defined all these measures.

The infants studied by Porter were assigned randomly to either a control or an experimental group. Both groups were pretested on the six measures, after which the infants in the experimental group were placed on a planned regimen of passive cycling exercise for a period of two months. Both groups were retested on the six measures at midpoint and at the end of the experiment. Since great care was taken to ensure that the only difference in the care given the infants in the two groups was the introduction of the independent variable, passive cycling exercises, it could reasonably be expected that the significantly greater gains in growth and development in the experimental group would be due to the introduction of this variable.

Not all experimental research follows the "true" experimental design. Campbell and Stanley (1963, pp. 6-27) have discussed six designs, three of which they called "preexperimental" designs, and three "true" designs. The former include no controls, while the latter provide for control groups. The preexperimental design used in a study by Valadez and Anderson (1972), in which a group of nurses was tested before and after attending a rehabilitation workshop, is known as the one-group pretest-posttest design.

THE HISTORICAL STUDY DESIGN

Although nurses have produced fewer historical studies than descriptive or experimental ones, interest in this type of inquiry is growing, particularly among doctoral candidates, who are increasingly basing their dissertations on historical research. The recent establishment of a national Nursing Archive within the Mugar Library at Boston University is also an indication of this growing interest.*

In contrast to descriptive research, which is present-oriented, and experimental research, which is predictive or future-oriented, historical research is oriented to the past. Nevertheless, it is also a scientific search for truth and makes use of careful methods of collecting and analyzing data.

Your purpose in doing a historical study will dictate the design for it. One cannot observe the events of the past or set up an experiment to discover truths about past events. The research method will need to be documentary and will make use of such sources as manuscripts, official records, laws, letters, minutes of meetings, eyewitness accounts, newspaper accounts, diaries, biographies, memoirs, and oral histories on tapes or films.

All documents must be carefully evaluated for their authenticity, and primary sources must be distinguished from secondary sources. A *primary source,* published or unpublished, is one that gives direct evidence; for example, a letter that describes the philosophy or point of view of the letter

*This data bank of nursing history is an integral part of Boston University's Division of Special Collections. The Nursing Archive is made up of collections of personal and institutional papers, histories of schools of nursing, and early publications related to nursing. The Archive is the official depository of the American Nurses' Association; the American Journal of Nursing Company's historical collection; the Nursing Education Funds, Inc., materials; and materials from the American Association of Colleges of Nursing. As of 1973, there were 85 manuscript collections and approximately 1,500 books. The materials are maintained under optimal conditions, and the retrieval system makes them readily available to scholars.

writer himself is a primary source. A *secondary source* is a report that is one or more steps removed from the actual event described; if it is all you can find, you should look for several other secondary sources in order to verify the data to the extent possible. However, even though you find corroborating evidence, your interpretations will have to remain guarded.* The search for original materials may involve real detective work and be quite time-consuming, but the experience of finding just the right material after much digging and searching is very satisfying.

The data found in a historical search must be evaluated for genuineness and relevance to the study in hand. It must be subjected to both external and internal criticism. *External criticism* involves asking whether the material is what it purports to be as to authorship, dates, and so forth. For example, was the letter you located really written by the person you are interested in? Sometimes letters are not dated, so the date will need to be established in some way. Or, you may know to whom the letter was sent, but not the name of the sender. "Research into Things Past; Tracking Down One of Miss Nightingale's Correspondents" is an interesting account of methods used in tracing the recipient of a series of letters (Monteiro, 1972).

After the letter, or other document has been authenticated, it may be subjected to *internal criticism* to determine the accuracy of the statements contained in it.

Finally, the document must be examined for its relevance to the investigation. It may be an authentic primary source,

---

*For examples of the use of the historical method and methods of documentation, see Austin's *Woolsey Sisters of New York, 1860–1900* (1971) and Roberts' *American Nursing: History and Interpretation* (1954).

but if it does not relate to your inquiry you cannot use it, no matter how interesting it is. Also, remember to examine the document in the context in which it was written or used. An understanding of the period in which it appeared is very important. Do not try to interpret or evaluate yesterday's documents by today's standards.

Historical research can be a most fascinating adventure. If you are interested in undertaking such a study, see Austin's (1958) article "The Historical Method in Nursing." It contains suggestions and ideas about kinds of historical studies that might be undertaken as well as the author's own views on the subject.

SUMMARY

In this chapter we have endeavored to show how one's research purpose helps in selecting a research design. We have also discussed three research methods most commonly employed in nursing research: descriptive or survey, experimental or explanatory, and historical or documentary. A variety of data collection methods used in research are presented in the next chapter, in which we also discuss the selection of a study sample.

REFERENCES

Austin, Anne L. The historical method in nursing. *Nurs Res* 7:4–10, Feb. 1958.
———. *The Woolsey Sisters of New York, 1860–1900.* Philadelphia, American Philosophical Society, 1971.
Campbell, Donald T. and Stanley, Julian C. *Experimental and*

Quasi-Experimental Designs for Research. Chicago, Rand Mc-Nally and Company, 1963.

Daly, Mary McDermed and Carr, John E. Tactile contact: a measure of therapeutic progress. *Nurs Res* 16:16–21, Winter 1967.

Dawson, Norma and Stern, Martha. Perceptions of priorities for home nursing care. *Nurs Res* 22:145–148, Mar.-Apr. 1973.

Fox, David J. *Fundamentals of Research in Nursing.* 2nd ed. New York, Appleton-Century-Crofts, 1970.

Golub, Sharon and Reznikoff, Marvin. Attitudes toward death: a comparison of nursing students and graduate nurses. *Nurs. Res* 20:503–508, Nov.-Dec. 1971.

Hulicka, Irene H. and Hulicka, Karel. To design experimental research. *Am J Nurs* 62:100–103, Feb. 1962.

Lindeman, Carol A. and Van Aernam, Betty. Nursing intervention with the presurgical patient—the effects of structured and unstructured preoperative teaching. *Nurs Res* 20:319–332, July-Aug. 1971.

Monteiro, Lois. Research into things past: tracking down one of Miss Nightingale's correspondents. *Nurs Res* 21:526–529, Nov.-Dec. 1972.

Porter, Luz S. The impact of physical-physiological activity on infants' growth and development. *Nurs Res* 21:210–219, May-June 1972.

Richards, Mary Ann Bruegel. A study of differences in psychological characteristics of students graduating from three types of basic nursing programs. *Nurs Res* 21:258–261, May-June 1972.

Roberts, Mary M. *American Nursing: History and Interpretation.* New York, Macmillan Company, 1954.

Valadez, Ana M. and Anderson, Elizabeth T. Rehabilitation workshops: change in attitudes in nurses. *Nurs Res* 21:132–137, Mar.-Apr. 1972.

Wilcox, Jane. Observer factors in the measurement of blood pressure. *Nurs Res* 10:4–17, Winter 1961.

Williams, Anne. A study of factors contributing to skin breakdown. *Nurs Res* 21:238–243, May-June 1972.

7

DATA COLLECTION

After the investigator has defined her purpose, stated her hypothesis, and determined her design or method, the next logical steps involve the choice of a method for collecting data and for selecting and developing a tool that will be used to collect the data. At the same time, thought must be given to the study population, commonly known as the *sample*.

METHODS OF COLLECTING DATA

Your reading of research reports in the nursing literature has undoubtedly made you aware of a variety of methods of collecting data. Those most commonly used in nursing research are: observation, the interview, the questionnaire, critical incidents, Q-sorts, diaries, record analyses, and nursing activity analyses.

All investigators use at least one and sometimes two or more of these methods. For example, Waters et al. (1972), in their exploratory study of technical and professional nursing, used both observation and the interview. They wanted to observe the decision-making behavior of nurses doing two types of nursing, but they also wanted to validate their observations through an interview with each of the nurses. That is, they wanted to substantiate the decision-making or problem-solving action of the nurse as it was observed and to collect further data on her thought processes related to her actions. Therefore, in addition to observing the nurse for a selected period of time, the observer met the observee as soon as she could after the observation period was over and interviewed her about the observed action.

Observation

Observation alone, or in combination with another method such as the interview or the questionnaire, is frequently used in nursing research. Observers may be disguised or undisguised, or they may have characteristics of both these types. Pearsall (1965) defined four types of observer: complete observer, observer-as-participant, participant-as-observer, and complete participant. The complete observer may be disguised or undisguised. For example, the investigator may observe behavior through a two-way mirror while those observed are completely unaware of her presence. Of course, this kind of observation does not influence the behavior of the subjects, since they are unaware of the fact that they are being observed. However, this method raises ethical questions that the investigator must answer.

Most commonly, the observer is known to the subjects. This was the case in the Waters et al. (1972) study. Each staff nurse to be observed was told why the observations were being made and was asked to participate. A major handicap that arises in this kind of observation is the result of the influence of the observer on the observed; it is generally conceded that subjects tend to try to help the researcher by behaving as they believe the researcher wants them to. Waters and her co-workers attempted to guard against this unwanted behavior by telling the subjects only part of the purpose; i.e., they were told only that their thought processes in making patient care decisions were being studied. What they were not told was that the observers would make comparisons between professional and technical nurses in relation to this decision making. Subjects in each of the two groups of nurses were given the same information, and it was thought that the observer's influence would be the same on all participants in the study.

A completely different type of observer, one who becomes a complete participant in the study, may or may not be recognized as an observer. For example, when nurses working on a unit are used as observers they are accepted as a natural part of the environment and can collect data without patients' becoming aware that they are being observed. The Brink (1972) study of heroin addicts exemplifiies this kind of observation; the study nurses on the unit made all the observations necessary for obtaining data on each patient. Another example of participant observation was described by Byerly (1969). She discussed this role of participant observer in relation to anthropological studies wherein the investigator becomes a part of the situation under study. Byerly explained the objectivity-subjectivity, scientific-integrity, and intervention-nonintervention aspects of participant observation. Of particular interest was her discussion of the attempts of the subjects to identify or define the role of the observer and their further attempts to make the observer "one of them" and to use her to achieve policy changes they wanted. Ragucci, also a nurse anthropologist, has discussed the nature of the participant observer in an article on the use of the ethnographic approach—a way of studying behavior in the natural setting. She described some of the approaches she used in establishing herself in an Italian-American enclave to study the health attitudes of the women living there and some of her experiences in collecting data during her 15-month stay in the enclave (Ragucci, 1972).

One of the major problems encountered by the participant observer is that it is difficult for nurse researchers observing nursing care to maintain objectivity and nonintervention.

The Interview

In studies in which the investigator is interested in obtaining facts, ideas, impressions, or opinions from the study subjects, and when it is possible for him, or his assistants, to be in personal contact with the study subjects, he may elect to use the interview method of data collection.

Interviews are of two types—structured and unstructured. The type used will depend on the researcher's purpose in using the interview method of gathering data. The *structured interview* is somewhat akin to the questionnaire in that each interview follows a set pattern of questioning. The data obtained are more objective than those obtained in the less formalized *unstructured interview,* which uses the open-end type of question in order to obtain freer responses. Such responses are more difficult to analyze than those obtained in a structured interview; their content must be analyzed by experts according to preestablished identification of the categories. In the Waters et al. study (1972), the responses were categorized under three areas that corresponded to the researchers' interests: (1) decision making, (2) scope of practice, and (3) attitude toward practice. The responses were also judged as to whether the action taken was technical or professional. Definitions of decision making, scope of practice, attitude toward practice, and technical and professional practice were developed from the literature in advance of the interviews. The categorizations and judgments of the responses were made independently by two expert judges who were not the interviewers. The findings were based only on those examples in which there was complete agreement between the two judges. This kind of planning and use of judges helps to ensure the validity and reliability of the content analysis.

The structured interview can be more objectively and easily tabulated. However, questions used must be carefully chosen to obtain the data needed. As mentioned earlier, the questions asked in interviews are similar to those included in questionnaires, but the data are collected in person; this also allows for some probing when the answers to questions are not clearly understood at first.

The Questionnaire

The questionnaire is a paper-and-pencil approach to the collection of data. Its advantage over the interview is that it can be used with subjects at a distance without greatly increasing the cost and time involved. It is most useful in surveys of large groups of people. The United States government's population census is a good example of the use of the questionnaire to survey a large number of people over a wide area.

Questionnaires may be employed to obtain demographic data, that is, social or vital statistics such as age, sex, marital status, educational background, etc. They can also be used to obtain information about certain types of phenomena; for example, Dammann (1972) used a questionnaire to determine the extent to which the curriculums of schools of nursing and schools of social work included information about the interprofessional aspects of their work. She mailed the questionnaire to all accredited schools of social work and to all schools of nursing accredited by the National League for Nursing.

Another investigator who used a questionnaire in survey research was Glass (1971). This investigator studied the use of the abstracts that are published in *Nursing Research*. Her questionnaire was mailed to a representative national sample of nurses she thought would be most likely to be readers of the abstracts—individual subscribers to *Nursing Research,* members of the National League for Nursing's Council of Baccalaureate and Higher Degree Programs, and members of the Public Health Nursing Section of the American Public Health Association.

In addition to descriptive data about phenomena such as that collected by Dammann and Glass, information about opinions, interests, and attitudes can also be sought by questionnaire. A questionnaire aimed at determining attitudes was used by Golub and Reznikoff (1971) to compare nursing students' and graduate nurses' attitudes toward death. They used six multiple-choice questions from a previously tested questionnaire. The questions were related to psychological factors, terminal illness, autopsy, suicide prevention, life maintenance efforts, and heart transplant.

The questions used can be either: (1) closed—for example, true-false or answerable by "yes" or "no"; or (2) open-ended. Answers obtained by open-end questions, like those obtained by unstructured interviews, are somewhat more difficult to analyze than those obtained by closed questions. The multiple-choice type as used by Golub and Reznikoff is a form of the closed question. Some questionnaires contain both closed and open-end questions, the latter being included for the purpose of obtaining a freer response. The purpose in using the questionnaire will help the investigator select the type of questions to use.

Success in using the questionnaire depends upon how carefully it is constructed. First, the questions should cover the significant areas to be studied. Thus, a good questionnaire is based on previous study. Either the questions have already been tested in previous research, as they were in the Dammann study, or they are based on careful observation, experience, consultation with experts, and systematic review of the literature. Second, the questions should be worded as carefully as possible to ensure understanding. *The Art of Asking Questions* (Payne, 1951) is a good source of information about phrasing questions. Third, the questions should be pretested on a group that is similar to but not the same as the sample you plan to study. The importance of this pretesting cannot be overemphasized. It should always be done unless the questions you plan to use have already been successfully tested in previous research and found to be valid and reliable.

One of the limitations of the questionnaire is the fact that not all individuals in the sample you select will return the questionnaire, and some of those who do return it will not answer all the questions, making their responses useless. Another limitation lies in the difficulty of constructing questions that will be interpreted in the same way by all the respondents. Furthermore, there may be a tendency on the part of the respondents to give answers they think are wanted. Keeping the respondent anonymous by asking him not to sign the questionnaire will help avoid this latter problem to some extent. Of course, questionnaires should always be accompanied by a stamped, addressed return envelope.

The Critical Incident Technique

The *critical incident technique* for obtaining data involves the use of written reports that describe previous experiences or observations (see Flanagan, 1954). These reports are based on the subject's memory of incidents that involved human activities. The activity described must be sufficiently complete in itself to illustrate the behavior under study. The incident as written by the subject is analyzed in terms of content categories developed by the investigator. Again, categorization of the material is more objective when done by independent expert judges other than the investigator.

Two examples of the use of the critical incident technique are Barham's (1965) study of nursing instructor behavior and Davitz's (1972) study of stressful situations in a Nigerian school of nursing. Barham asked directors, instructors, and nursing students to describe one example of ineffective teaching behavior and one example of effective teaching behavior; these were categorized by the investigator, and two judges independently validated the categorizations. Davitz asked students to write about their stressful experiences during training; two coders independently rated the incidents and coded them under the following categories: academic, personal, social, and clinical experience.

The Q-Sort Technique

The *Q-sort technique* has been used at times in nursing research. Whiting (1955) described its use in studying interpersonal relationships in nursing. He suggested that the Q-sort could best be used in nursing research to: (1) compare attitudes or opinions of different persons or groups, and (2) determine a change in attitude or opinion of individuals or groups over time.

The Q-sort consists of a set of cards on each of which a statement is printed. The subject is asked to sort the cards into a specified number of piles according to the importance of the statement. In the Whiting study there were 100 statements on nurse-patient relationships. The task was to arrange these statements into nine piles, and the number of cards put in each pile was to be as follows:

$$1 \quad 4 \quad 11 \quad 21 \quad 26 \quad 21 \quad 11 \quad 4 \quad 1$$

This arrangement is known as a *forced-choice arrangement*. From left to right, the piles are numbered one through nine; the subject is told to put the card with the statement he thinks is most important in the first pile, the four next most important ones in the second pile, and so on. The card with the statement considered least important goes on the last, or ninth, pile. The final sort resembles the normal distribution (see chapter 8, p. 90).

Another, more recent, study in which the Q-sort was used was that by Brophy (1971) on relationships among self-role congruences and nursing experience. Brophy used the Hanlon Q-sort to obtain real and ideal self-concepts of the subjects and their perceptions of the ideal nurse role. This Q-sort consisted of 50 statements to be placed in a forced-choice distribution of nine categories from "most like me" to "most unlike me."

The Q-sort is usually a difficult task for the subject. However, the job can be made easier if directions are carefully given and if the subject understands the importance of the study. If you plan to use this technique, the articles by Whiting and Brophy, as well as some of the references these two authors list, will be most helpful to you.

Other Techniques

In addition to the major data collection techniques we have been discussing, several other techniques are available. Such nursing records as nurses' notes and Kardexes are commonly used in both ongoing and retrospective research. The Brink (1972) study of heroin addicts made use of nurses' records. The use of records presents problems, however, since errors and omissions occur in recording, as is well known. Some of these errors can be overcome in ongoing research by careful preparation of the nurses doing the recording. In retrospective or historical research no control can be exercised, and the investigator must use what is there and verify it in other ways, such as by comparison with other contemporary records.

Field-work notes or diaries are also used in collecting data. Anthropologists, for example, use them when studying the cultures of groups of people. This special kind of recording focuses on the investigator's specific area of interest. You will find a discussion of the use of field-work notes in "The Purpose and Credibility of Qualitative Research" (Glaser and Strauss, 1966).

Finally, a data collection technique that has been used in nursing studies for a number of years is the nursing activity analysis. This technique has been considered more helpful in problem solving than in actual research. The purpose of studies using this method is to determine how nursing personnel spend their time, and particularly how this time is divided between patient care and other unit activities. The method is described in detail in the government publication *How to Study Nursing Activities in a Patient Unit* (U.S. Department of Health, Education and Welfare, 1964).

A glance through several issues of *Nursing Research* will give some indication of the variety of tools used in research. Some are used to collect data, others to record data that have been collected. Some of those used to collect data are also the recording instruments. For example, subjects may be asked to complete a checklist which, of course, may also serve as the record of the data obtained. For her study "Importance of Selected Nursing Activities," White (1972) used a checklist consisting of 50 nursing activities which the subjects (nurses and their patients) checked according to whether they considered the activity to be of extreme importance, very important, of medium importance, of slight importance, of no importance, or not applicable.

Although tools used to record observations are often of the checklist variety, other possible tools are printouts of monitoring systems, videotapes, diaries, and field-work notes. The questionnaire, of course, may also be considered a tool for collecting and recording data.

Reports in the January-February 1972 issue of *Nursing Research* describe such other tools as the electrocardiogram (Segall, 1972), the tape recorder (Benner and Kramer, 1972), a behavior rating scale (Brink, 1972), a telephone lecture network system (Kellberg, 1972), and thermometers (Nichols, et al., 1972).

Other data-collecting tools that have been used include paper-and-pencil tests, attitude and anxiety scales, physiological tests (e.g., urinalyses), closed circuit television, electronic monitoring machines, x-ray equipment, and sphygmomanometers. An interesting new tool used in the study of decubitus ulcers, thermography, has been reported by Verhonick et al. (1972). In this technique the infrared energy of the skin is measured. The thermogram, or thermal picture, shows gradations of skin temperature which indirectly reflect the pressure on the area.

These are a few of the tools in current use. You may be able to locate others in the research literature or even think of some yourself.

Whatever method is used to collect and record data, it should be so constructed that different persons using the same tool will obtain the same kind of data. Observer reliability checks and the use of independent judges are two ways of assuring this. In addition, in experimental studies you must make sure that the observers used do not know which subjects are the controls and which are in the experimental group.

VALIDITY AND RELIABILITY OF DATA-COLLECTING INSTRUMENTS

In the foregoing discussion of methods of collecting and recording data, the words "validity" and "reliability" were frequently used, since an evaluation of research findings requires that the validity and reliability of the tool may be established.

The *validity* of a research tool refers to its ability to obtain the needed data. It tells the investigator whether the tool will measure what she wants it to measure. The term *face validity* is sometimes used to indicate that validity has been established simply by looking at a tool—a questionnaire or checklist, for example—to see whether the items are the important ones to be included.

A better way to test the measuring ability of a tool is to establish its *content validity*. To do this, the investigator points out the authority for the use of the content in the questions, checklist, or other type of tool. This authority may be derived from the literature, from the investigator's personal observations, or from consultation with others who are experts on the content involved.

A still better but more complex method of testing validity involves testing results on the instrument with results from the use of another known instrument that tests the same sort of content. For example, if you are testing for evidence of anxiety and you can find a *valid* test of anxiety, you can then give both tests to a group and compare the results. This will provide you with a measure of the validity of your tool in comparison with one that has been validated in previous investigations.

The *reliability* of a tool indicates its accuracy with respect to stability and repeatability in collecting data. In a paper-and-pencil test, for example, a test-retest method is commonly used to determine the test's reliability. That is, the test is given to a group similar to the group that will be studied and, some time later, the test is readministered to the same group. Sufficient time must elapse between testing so that the memory of the test items is not fresh in the subjects' minds. If the test results remain the same or similar to those obtained the first time, the test is considered reliable. In other words, the reliability of an instrument is related to its ability to obtain the same data when repeated.

Other methods of testing reliability include the alternate form test and the split-half or odd-even test of reliability. In the alternate form test, a two-part test with each part containing similar questions is devised and administered to a group. To prove reliability, the subjects must give similar answers in both parts of the test; in other words, one looks at the correlation of scores obtained from the two sets of questions. The split-half test for reliability involves only one set of questions, but two scores are obtained for comparison, one for the first half of the questions and one for the second half. The odd-even method also involves the use of two scores, but in this instance one is obtained from the answers to the odd-numbered questions and one from answers to the even-numbered questions.

Barham's (1965) report of her study using the critical incident technique described her tests for validity and reliability in some detail. You may want to look at this report as well as several others to see how other investigators have tested the research tools they used for validity and reliability. Frequently the tool to be used is tested in a pilot study, an important step in the development of a new tool. We suggest that, whenever possible, the novice researcher locate and use a tool—or a modification of one—that is already in existence and known to be valid.

THE SAMPLE

A very important step in data collection is the selection of the sample, which is a representative selection of the group of the population to be studied. The sample must be consistent with the problem to be studied. For example, if one wishes to compare the attitudes of practicing nurses and physicians toward the use of clinical nurse specialists, the sample must consist of both nurses and doctors; one could not use a sample of just nurses or just physicians, or a sample of nursing students and interns.

In addition, all characteristics to be studied must be represented in the sample. For example, in her study of coronary care nurses, Kellberg (1972) wanted to study nurses working on all three shifts in coronary care units; therefore, it was necessary for her sample to include nurses who worked on all three shifts. The study of rectal thermometer placement times for febrile adults, by Nichols et al. (1972), included an equal number of men and women patients whose rectal temperatures ranged from 100.6°F to 104°F. The sample in Brink's (1972) exploratory study of behavioral characteristics of heroin addicts on a short-term detoxification program consisted of 42 addicts admitted to one psychiatric ward for detoxification during the five-month study period. The addicts included both male and female patients. Glass was interested in obtaining a sample representative of users and nonusers of abstracts. Therefore, in her study *"Nursing Research Abstracts:* A Users' Study" (1971), she utilized a national sample that included respondents from different professional, institutional, and geographic settings. The sample also represented nurses most likely to be potential users of the abstracts. She drew her sample from the list of individual subscribers to *Nursing Research* and from the membership lists of the Council of Baccalaureate and Higher Degree Programs of the National League for Nursing and of the Public Health Nursing Section of the American Public Health Association.

The sample must also be representative of the total population of the group under study. Since it is frequently not possible to study the total population of, say, heroin addicts on all detoxification units, one settles for all the patients—or a sample of them—in one institution or in a group of institutions. If the sample is sufficiently large, it is assumed that the characteristics or phenomena observed will be representative of those that would be found in other groups. Replications of the same study in other institutions and in other parts of the country will establish representativeness.

Most current clinical research in nursing is limited to small, though representative, samples; therefore, generalizations to the total population can only be tentative.

When the investigator plans to test a hypothesis by using a statistical analysis of his data, he selects what is known as a *random sample;* that is, everyone in the group from which the sample is taken must have an equal chance or probability of being selected. In this chapter we have mentioned two studies in which random sampling was used: (1) Kellberg's (1972) study of coronary care nurses, which utilized a random sample of nurses in both coronary care units and other units; and (2) Brophy's (1971) study of relationships among self-role congruences and nursing experience, in which a random sample of 60 nurses from a staff of 125 in one general hospital was employed.

A *stratified random sample* refers to a sample that has been randomized according to some added factor or factors such as age, educational background, type of school, or perhaps religious affiliation. For example, in a study of nursing students one may want to use a random sample in which the number of students is divided among representatives of diploma, associate degree, and baccalaureate programs.

A random sample can be obtained by putting slips containing the names of all possible subjects in a container, shaking the container well, and then withdrawing the required number of slips, one at a time. In order for this procedure to produce a truly random sample, each time a name is selected, the slip is replaced in the container; if it comes up a second time, it is simply replaced again and another one drawn. In this way, every subject has an equal chance on each draw. Another method of making a random selection is to use a table of random numbers. (Tables of random numbers and explanations of their uses can be found in any standard text on statistics.)

SUMMARY

This chapter has presented information about a most important aspect of research—data collection. We have described a number of common methods of collecting data, methods of testing the validity and reliability of the instruments used in collecting and recording data, and the selection of an appropriate sample. Throughout this discussion, objectivity or freedom from bias is stressed. The next step in the research process, analyzing the collected data, will be presented in the following chapter.

REFERENCES

Barham, Virginia Z. Identifying effective behavior of the nursing instructor through critical incidents. *Nurs Res* 14:65–69, Winter 1965.

Benner, Patricia and Kramer, Marlene. Role conceptions and integrative role behavior of nurses in special care and regular hospital nursing units. *Nurs Res* 21:20–29, Jan.-Feb. 1972.

Brink, Pamela J. Behavioral characteristics of heroin addicts on a short-term detoxification program. *Nurs Res* 21:38–45, Jan.-Feb. 1972.

Brophy, Elizabeth B. Relationships among self-role congruences and nursing experience. *Nurs Res* 20:447–450, Sept.-Oct. 1971.

Byerly, Elizabeth Lee. The nurse researcher as participant-observer in a nursing setting. *Nurs Res* 18:230–236, May-June 1969.

Dammann, Gloria L. A. Interprofessional aspects of nursing and social work curricula. *Nurs Res* 21:160–163, Mar.-Apr. 1972.

Davitz, Lois Jean. Identification of stressful situations in a Nigerian school of nursing. *Nurs Res* 21:352–357, July-Aug. 1972.

Flanagan, John C. The critical incident technique. *Psychological Bulletin,* 51:327–358, July 1954.

Glaser, Barney G. and Strauss, Anselm L. The purpose and credibility of qualitative research. *Nurs Res* 15:56–61, Winter 1966.

Glass, Leah. *Nursing Research* abstracts: a users' study. *Nurs Res* 20:152–158, Mar.-Apr. 1971.

Golub, Sharon and Reznikoff, Marvin. Attitudes toward death: a comparison of nursing students and graduate nurses. *Nurs Res* 20:503–508, Nov.-Dec. 1971.

Kellberg, Elsa R. Coronary care nurse profile. *Nurs Res* 21:30–37, Jan.-Feb. 1972.

Nichols, Glennadee A.; Kucha, Deloros H.; and Mahoney, Rosemarie P. Rectal thermometer placement times for febrile adults. *Nurs Res* 21:76–77, Jan.-Feb. 1972.

Payne, Stanley. *The Art of Asking Questions.* Princeton, New Jersey, Princeton University Press, 1951.

Pearsall, Lillian. Participant observation as role and method in behavioral research. *Nurs Res* 14:37–42, Winter 1965.

Ragucci, Antoinette T. Approaches to the study of nursing questions and the development of nursing science. The ethnographic approach and nursing research. *Nurs Res* 21:485–490, Nov.-Dec. 1972.

Segall, Mary E. Cardiac responsivity to auditory stimulation in premature infants. *Nurs Res* 21:15–19, Jan.-Feb. 1972.

U.S. Department of Health, Education and Welfare. Public Health Service. Division of Nursing. *How to Study Nursing Activities in a Patient Unit.* Revised. Public Health Service Publication No. 370. Washington, D.C., Government Printing Office, 1964.

Verhonick, Phyllis J.; Lewis, David W.; and Goller, Herbert O. Thermography in the study of decubitus ulcers. *Nurs Res* 21:233–237, May-June 1972.

Waters, Verle H.; Chater, Shirley S.; Vivier, Mary L.; Urrea, Judithe H.; and Wilson, Holly S. Technical and professional nursing: an exploratory study. *Nurs Res* 21:124–131, Mar.-Apr. 1972.

White, Marguerite B. Importance of selected nursing activities. *Nurs Res* 21:4–14, Jan.-Feb. 1972.

Whiting, J. Frank. Q-Sort: a technique for evaluating perceptions of interpersonal relationships. *Nurs Res* 4:70–73, 1955.

8

ANALYSIS OF THE DATA

For an investigator to make a meaningful analysis of the data collected in a study, the methods used to collect it must be appropriate to the study of the problem being investigated. For example, in the Brink (1972) study of the behavioral characteristics of heroin addicts, the method used for collecting data was observation, and the tools used were patient records and a rating scale. The sample consisted of patients admitted to the short-term detoxification unit in one hospital. In her original plan, Brink not only selected the sample and the data collection method but she also indicated that she would use a method of data analysis that could be related to the problem she studied. The method of analyzing data that is selected for a study involves knowing in advance how the data are to be summarized and interpreted.

There are three very simple reasons why the investigator must think through what her method of analysis will be at the time she decides on her method of collecting data; she must determine: (1) what data she will need to collect; (2) how she can collect it; and (3) whether she can collect it at all. For example, in the Brink study the data to be collected were to consist of demographic and quantitative descriptions of certain facts related to the subjects' age, race, sex, occupation, education, employment, and religion. Brink also wanted to determine specific facts (by hospital shift) about the addicts' habits and lengths of hospitalization and about types as well as units of medication given. Ratings of behavior were to be examined in light of these variables. Therefore, all the variables had to be determined in advance so that data on them would be available for the kind of analysis the investigator had planned. The beginning investigator who does not study the situation carefully enough during the planning stage can find, when she comes to the stage of analysis, that she has not collected some of the information she needs. There is no question about it: the more time spent in planning all phases of the study, the better the chances of ending up with a well-designed study.

CLASSIFYING AND ORGANIZING THE DATA

Once data are collected, they must be organized and displayed in a fashion that will help the researcher to understand them. One can begin by grouping like facts together. If the data include scores of a group on a test, they can be tallied somewhat as follows:

Scores	Tally	Totals
100		
99	I	1
98		
97	II	2
96		
95	‖‖	5
etc.		

In other words, having like scores grouped together gives one a clearer, more concise picture of the data.

The data for a research study may be either qualitative or quantitative. The Davitz (1972) study, mentioned in chapter 7, used the critical incident method of collecting qualitative data. In that study, *content analysis categories,* i.e., appropriate subject headings or classifications, were established, and two coders independently classified the content in the reported incidents according to these categories. Their findings were recorded in simple numerical frequencies (Davitz, 1972, p. 354).

The data collected in the Brink study were mainly quantitative in nature. Some of the data were *nominal, that is,* names, (age, sex, race); some were *ordinal, that is, numbers* or rank order (numbers of patients for whom drugs were ordered and rankings of patient behaviors). The data, which had been collected one by one on checklists or from the patients' records, were grouped to facilitate analysis of their meaning and presented in tabular form. Some of Brink's data were grouped by percentages and some by rank order, as shown in Examples 1 and 2, tables taken from her study.

Example 1. Data Grouped by Percentages

TABLE 2. *Number and Percentage of Patients by Sex with Drugs Ordered*

	Methadone		Soma		Pro-Banthine		Valium and/or Compazine		Sleeping Medications	
Patients	N	%	N	%	N	%	N	%	N	%
Male	27	100	9	33	4	15	21	77	22	81
Female	15	100	10	66	6	40	11	73	14	93
Total	42	100	19	45	10	24	32	77	36	85

Source: Brink, Pamela J. Behavioral characteristics of heroin addicts on a short-term detoxification program. *Nurs Res* 21:41, Jan.-Feb. 1972. Copyright by American Journal of Nursing Company and reprinted with their permission.

Example 2.   Data Grouped by Rank Order

TABLE 5.   *Rank Order of Behavioral Acts for Male and Female Addicts during Hospitalization*

Behaviors	Males Rank Order	Males Scale Value	Females Rank Order	Females Scale Value
Sedentary activities	1	25	1	25
Retired after midnight	2	18	5	12
Active activities	3	13	16	4
Drowsy during the day	4	12	4	13
Slept at intervals during the night	5	10	6	12
Slept late in the morning	6	10	11	7
Listless and apathetic	7	9	3	14
Questions when medications are due	8	9	8	11
No breakfast	9	8	2	15
Restless sleep	10	8	9	11
Awake during the night	11	6	7	12
Irritable if medications not given on request	12	6	13	7
Angry at staff	13	5	10	9
Requests medications when the staff is busy	14	5	15	5
Questions nurses' judgment	15	5	12	7
Asleep during the day	16	4	17	4
Accuses staff of not giving medications	17	2	14	6
Threatens to leave against medical advice	18	1	20	1
Threatens to report nurses' behavior to the physician	19	1	21	1
Aggression to property	20	0	18	4
Angry at other patients	21	0	19	3

Source: Brink, Pamela J. Behavioral characteristics of heroin addicts on a short-term detoxification program. *Nurs Res* 21:43, Jan.-Feb. 1972. Copyright by American Journal of Nursing Company and reprinted with their permission.

As can be seen in Example 1, both actual numbers and percentages of patients observed by Brink for certain variables are given. This is a good procedure because it allows the reader to see at a glance what the percentages really mean. It is of the utmost importance that this procedure be adhered to when small numbers are involved. For instance, Example 1 shows that 40 percent of the female patients received Pro-Banthine, but this represented only 6 women. If one did not know the number, one might be unduly impressed with the percentage shown in the table.

Example 2 shows a method of ranking. In this instance, all patient behaviors were given a value on a predetermined scale. The average scale values for men and women on the 21 behaviors are shown in rank order, with the behavior having the highest scale value (25) receiving a rank of 1 and that having the lowest scale value receiving a rank of 21. On three of the behaviors, the men and the women in the study received the same rank; their ranks differed somewhat on the rest of the behaviors observed.

Most of the simple evaluative studies in which you may be involved will be descriptive and will require grouping of data by frequencies and percentages or rankings, whether by scores, tallies of questionnaire answers, or enumerations of observations made. In more complex descriptive studies and in experimental research, more sophisticated groupings may be made: for example, averages and mean scores rather than the actual scores may be grouped for analysis as was done in the study reported by Segall (1972, p. 17) on responses of premature infants to auditory stimulation (Examples 3 and 4).

Data that have been collected must be organized in some fashion so that they can be analyzed and so that the investigator can arrive at a statement of results. As we noted in the Brink study, data can be organized in a variety of ways for inspection and analysis in order to give the researcher as

Example 3.   Data Grouped by Mean Scores

TABLE 2.   *Mean Cardiac Scores to Female Voices for 30 Aroused Subjects Who Received Auditory Stimulation and 30 Aroused Subjects Who Did Not Receive Auditory Stimulation*

| | Mother's Voice | | | Unfamiliar Female Voice | | |
	Pre[a]	Peak[b]	Change[c]	Pre	Peak	Change
Experimental	192.70	168.17	—24.53	191.33	171.83	—19.50
Control	192.62	184.67	— 7.95	192.96	184.63	— 8.33

[a] Pre = Prestimulus level.
[b] Peak = Peak level.
[c] Change = Difference between prestimulus and peak levels.

Source: Segall, Mary E. Cardiac responsivity to auditory stimulation in premature infants. *Nurs Res* 21:17, Jan.-Feb. 1972. Copyright by American Journal of Nursing Company and reprinted with their permission.

much information as possible. Brink organized her data according to such variables as day of study, sex, age, type of activity, and type of medication.

The reason for organizing data for analysis is to make manifest possible relationships, proportions, trends, or tendencies; that is, to reveal the nature of the information that has been gathered. For example, there may be sex differences, or differences related to age. Brink found differences in the number of negative behavioral acts according to day of hospitalization. She also found a tendency for "the withdrawing heroin addict to be sedentary, participate in few activities, be drowsy during the day, and complain of constipation" (p. 45).

When data are presented in tabular form it is important that they be adequately and properly labeled. Each table should have a title that describes its contents and should be

Example 4. Data Grouped by Averages

FIGURE 1. *Reaction to White Noise by Two Groups of Premature Infants*

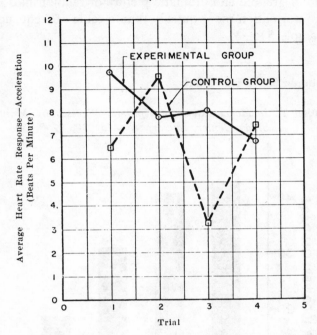

Source: Segall, Mary E. Cardiac responsivity to auditory stimulation in premature infants. *Nurs Res* 21:17, Jan.-Feb. 1972. Copyright by American Journal of Nursing Company and reprinted with their permission.

set up with both vertical and horizontal columns. Each row and column should have a heading that describes the information in the respective row or column. In the tables shown in this chapter the titles are descriptive of the table contents, and each row and column is carefully identified. (For a more detailed discussion of tables see Turabian (1973), pp. 159–171.)

Graphs and bar charts may be used to present data. This kind of graphic and dramatic picture of relationships will give the information more quickly than a table of frequencies (see Example 5).

Example 5. A Bar Chart

FIGURE 1. *Incidence Rates of Episodic Illnesses by Month, Child Study Center, January 15–May 29, 1968*

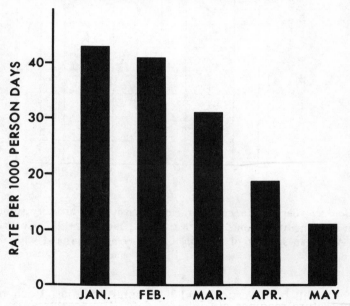

Source: MacCarthy, Jessie and Morrison, Joan. An explanatory test of a method of studying illness among preschool children. *Nurs Res* 21:323, July-Aug. 1972. Copyright by American Journal of Nursing Company and reprinted with their permission.

STATISTICAL ANALYSIS OF DATA

In addition to utilizing simple enumeration, grouping, and inspection in analyzing collected information, statistical analysis may be used. This includes such measures of central tendency as means, medians, modes, and standard deviation, as well as more sophisticated measures to estimate the chances that the findings can be generalized to the larger population.

If your study requires the use of statistics and you have not had special preparation in this area, you should consult a statistician about this phase of your study, and you should do this before you start to collect the data to make sure you know what statistics to use. You should also seek his help in computing the statistics, in analyzing the results of the computation, and in deciding on the correct method of reporting the findings.

Descriptive Statistics

Statistical analysis is commonly used in complex descriptive studies and in experimental research in which the findings on groups are compared. Statistics which describe data include some methods we have already mentioned: frequency distribution or grouping of the raw data, either nominal or ordinal, and interval data. *Interval data,* which we have not mentioned before, refer to data on a scale; for example, temperature readings are interval data. Temperatures can be 98.6, 98.7, 98.8, and so on, and are reported at the intervals noted, whereas ordinal data represent a count of something and would be reported as 98, 99, 100, and so on.

To describe data we may wish to show a range—for example, the range of scores on a test before and after some treatment or course. We may also want to show the mean, median, or mode, and the standard or average deviation from the mean.

The *range* is the distance between the top and bottom scores. The *mode* is the score that occurs most frequently. These two measures may be important to know, particularly if the distribution of scores is skewed in some way. The *median* is the exact middle score and is obtained by separating the scores into an upper and lower half. The *mean* is obtained by adding all the scores and dividing this sum by the total number of scores.

The *standard deviation* is a frequently used statistic that shows how scores will vary about the mean. The mean is a measure of central tendency, while the standard deviation is a measure of the variability of scores about the mean. Methods of computing the standard deviation can be found in any basic text on statistics. Example 6 shows the standard deviations for data which resemble the normal curve. When distribution is normal, most of the scores (68.2 percent) will

Example 6. The Normal Curve and Standard Deviations

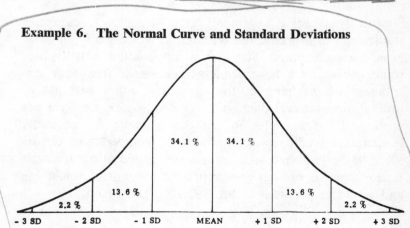

		34.1 %	34.1 %			
	13.6 %			13.6 %		
2.2 %					2.2 %	
- 3 SD	- 2 SD	- 1 SD	MEAN	+ 1 SD	+ 2 SD	+ 3 SD

fall between −1 and +1 standard deviation from the mean, and 95.4 percent will fall between −2 and +2 standard deviations.

Another way of showing relationships is through the use of correlation procedures. Correlations show either a positive or a negative relationship. A −1 relationship indicates a perfect negative relationship between two groups or variables studied, while a +1 indicates that they show a perfect positive relationship. That is, in the first case (−1), when one variable occurs, the other does not; in the second case (+1), when one occurs the other can be expected to occur also. A zero correlation indicates no relationship at all. Of course, there are graduations between −1, 0, and +1. These are always expressed as parts of 1; for example, .80, .70, .10, and so on.

Statistical Inference

In addition to the use of descriptive statistics, the investigator may use tests of significance when this is necessary to infer whether an observed difference is small and therefore not significant or large and therefore significant. For example, we might consider the study discussed in chapter 3, the comparison of effectiveness of two methods of teaching diabetic patients self-care—group instruction versus programmed instruction. If one found that the group having programmed instruction did better on the measurements used, one would want to know whether the difference in the data obtained was significant or merely due to chance. Two frequently used inferential statistics are the *chi-square* $(x)^2$ and the *t test*, although others are also used. Chi-square is used when the data collected on random samples consist of frequencies in discrete categories. It is a ratio—the sum of quotients obtained by dividing the square of the differences between the observed and theoretical or expected frequencies by the theoretical frequencies. The ratio is expressed as follows:

$$x^2 = \Sigma \; \frac{(fo - fe)^2}{fe}$$

$$\Sigma = \text{sum}$$
$$fo = \text{observed frequencies}$$
$$fe = \text{expected frequencies}$$

Chi-square can be used to analyze differences among groups compared on qualitative variables. An example of the use of x^2 can be seen in Berthold's study of "Nursing Research Grant Proposals: What Influenced Their Approval or Disapproval in Two National Granting Agencies" (1973). Her x^2 computations were based upon a 2 by 2 contingency table—approved–disapproved proposals by critical comments–no critical comments. (See Berthold, Table 2, p. 296.)

The t test may be used to test the differences between means of small samples which have been randomly selected. It is based on the t distribution, which is different from the normal distribution, i.e., the smaller the sample, the flatter the curve becomes with proportionally more cases distributed at the ends of the curve. The ratio for the t test has been expressed by Abdellah and Levine (1965, p. 712) as:

$$t = \frac{\text{difference in sample means minus difference in population means}}{\text{standard error of the difference in sample means}}$$

In this formula the difference between the means of the sample and the means of the population is divided by a quotient (standard error) obtained by dividing the standard deviation of the sample by the square root of the number in the sample. An example of the use of the *t* test to measure results can be seen in Table 4 of the Porter study mentioned in earlier chapters and entitled "The Impact of Physical-Psychological Activity on Infants' Growth and Development" (1972, p. 216), in which she presents the tests of significance of the difference between the 47 infants in the experimental group and the 47 in the control group on the selected variables— weight; height; motor, adaptive, language, and personal/social behavior—for the midtest and posttest periods.

Detailed explanation of how these and other tests are calculated, and when one is used rather than another, is beyond the purpose of this book and, again, you are referred to a basic text on statistics. However, it is important to understand what is meant by significant differences between sets of data and what the term "level of significance" means.

The *level of significance* refers to the probability that the difference between sets of data is due to chance. The investigator sets the probability level she will accept at the time she designs her research. For example, she may decide she will accept a probability (p) of .01. This $p = .01$ or $p < .01$ (which sets the probability at 1 percent or less than 1 percent) means that results would occur by chance less than 1 percent of the time, or only one time out of every 100 times. Acceptable levels of significance are usually .01 to .05. If the significant difference turns out to be greater than .05, say .10 or .20, there would be too great a probability that the difference observed was due to chance, and the investigator would report that there was no significant difference. These tests of significance are particularly useful in analyzing the data in relation to the hypothesis made at the beginning of the study. The null hypothesis, you will remember, states that no difference will be found. If a significant difference is found, the null hypothesis is rejected; if no significant difference is found, the null hypothesis is accepted.

Remember that the purpose of statistical analysis is to make possible the interpretation of collected data; it does not correct data that happen to be biased or that are based on inadequate or inappropriate samples. Moreover, nursing data which have been found to be highly significant statistically also need to be examined in terms of their clinical significance; that is, whether the findings are of any value to nursing.

SUMMARY

As a result of your inspection of the data, which you have organized and displayed in as many ways as were appropriate and which you have subjected to statistical analysis when this was indicated, you have been able to formulate a statement of your findings. Now you are ready to interpret the findings, draw conclusions, and consider the implications of these findings and conclusions.

REFERENCES

Abdellah, Faye and Levine, Eugene. *Better Patient Care through Nursing Research.* New York, The Macmillan Company, 1965.

Berthold, Jeanne S. Nursing research grant proposals: what influenced their approval or disapproval in two national granting agencies. *Nurs Res* 22:292–299, July-Aug. 1973.

Brink, Pamela J. Behavioral characteristics of heroin addicts on a short-term detoxification program. *Nurs Res* 21:38–45, Jan-Feb. 1972.

Davitz, Lois Jean. Identification of stressful situations in a Nigerian school of nursing. *Nurs Res* 21:352–357, July-Aug. 1972.

MacCarthy, Jessie and Morison, Joan. An explanatory test of a method of studying illness among preschool children. *Nurs Res* 21:319–326, July-Aug. 1972.

Porter, Luz S. The impact of physical-physiological activity on infants' growth and development. *Nurs Res* 21:210–219, May-June 1972.

Segall, Mary E. Cardiac responsivity to auditory stimulation in premature infants. *Nurs Res* 21:15–19, Jan-Feb. 1972.

Turabian, Kate L. *Manual for Writers of Term Papers, Theses, and Dissertations.* 4th ed. Chicago, University of Chicago Press, 1973.

9

FINDINGS, CONCLUSIONS,
AND RECOMMENDATIONS

Perhaps the admonition "be cautious" is the best advice that can be given to the beginning researcher who, having analyzed her data, has reached the point of discussing her findings, drawing some conclusions, and making some recommendations. While it is important for the investigator to point out and discuss some of the possible meanings of her findings as shown by that data, it is equally important that she avoid drawing conclusions that go beyond those indicated by the data and making recommendations that cannot be justified by the results of the study.

SOME EXAMPLES OF CONCLUSIONS
AND RECOMMENDATIONS

A study by Walker (1972) entitled "The Postsurgery Heart Patient: Amount of Uninterrupted Time for Sleep and Rest during the First, Second, and Third Postoperative Days in a Teaching Hospital" illustrates how one can discuss study findings in terms of limitations involved and yet make some suggestions about nursing care which are based on the findings. Walker pointed out (p. 169) the number of interruptions that occurred in the sleep and rest of the subjects during the time of her study. She recognized the limitations imposed by the small sample size and the limited number of observations made. Keeping these facts in mind, she went on to make suggestions that nurses might consider in their efforts to reduce the sleep interruptions of patients in coronary and intensive care units. She also suggested the need for additional studies of patterns of interactions of patients over a consecutive 24-hour period (her study covered an 8-hour period) and for periods beyond the first three postoperative days.

In the report of a study by Eisler, Wolfer, and Diers (1972), "Relationship between Need for Social Approval and Postoperative Recovery and Welfare," one sees again the objective reporting of results and, in addition, a discussion by the investigators which considers the possible limitations of the Social Desirability scale they used and the possible implications for further research.

The report of the Brink (1972) study, which we have frequently referred to in this book, also exemplifies careful reporting of findings and a cautious interpretation of the findings in terms of behavior nurses might look for in heroin addicts on a short-term detoxification program. Brink was careful to suggest that her findings might not necessarily apply to patients on a longer program.

You might find it profitable to look at the "findings" and "discussion" sections of other study reports, noting especially the use of such phrases as "results seem to indicate," "this finding suggests," and "possible explanations are," which reflect investigators' caution in reporting. Also note how the investigators relate findings to the purpose of the study and to the hypotheses made before the study began.

LIMITATIONS

Important limitations should always be recognized in the published report of any study. They may be simply implied, or they may be spelled out early in the report and repeated in the discussion of the findings. The Woods (1972) report of the study "Patterns of Sleep in Postcardiotomy Patients" included a special section on limitations. This illustrates the importance of describing the limitations early so they can be kept in mind when considering the data analysis and conclusions. In this case, Woods called attention to the small sample size, the limited number of observations, the possibility of observer error, and the existence of uncontrolled environmental factors such as noise. The investigator may not be able to control all the variables in the environment, but it is essential for her to recognize that other variables are present.

In another study, "Recovery Room Behavior and Postoperative Convalescence," Elms (1972) described limitations in her discussion of the findings:

> The present study did not, however, explore all the complexities of surgical adjustment. The postoperative interviews might not have reflected all important aspects of the patient's recovery. Certainly to quantify the patient's feelings was difficult; the scores obtained were only relative and not absolute measures. Although the study used a diverse population through random selection of patients, expanded and quantified the observational categories for recovery room behavior, and systematically evaluated certain aspects of postoperative convalescence, it by no means exhausted the possibility for further study (p. 396).

The most common limitations in clinical nursing studies are: (1) small sample size and unrepresentativeness of the sample; for example, a small convenience sample in one or two hospitals; and (2) the use of relatively untested tools for gathering data, that is, schedules or questionnaires which the investigator developed for a study but which had not been adequately tested for validity and reliability. This is not meant to suggest that small clinical studies should not be done, but only that the limitations should be explicitly recognized. In fact, one outcome of small studies may be ideas and hypotheses for larger, more sophisticated studies.

RELATING CONCLUSIONS TO THE PURPOSE OF THE STUDY

It is very important for the investigator to remember that the conclusions reached in a study must be related to the purpose, hypothesis, and results of the data analysis. For example, Elms reported that her findings suggested:

> that patients who had a relatively high percentage of negative responses to stimuli in the recovery room environment tended to have more difficulty during their convalescence in the hospital, but that other aspects of recovery-room behavior were not consistently associated with measures of later convalescence. Therefore, the hypothesis that behavior in the recovery room predicts postoperative convalescence was only partially confirmed (p. 396).

A look at other studies mentioned in this chapter (those by Woods, Walker, Brink, and Eisler et al.) will show that the investigators' conclusions and recommendations were consistent with the stated purposes or hypotheses of the studies as well as with the method of study and the findings. For example, the purposes in the Woods study were:

> to ascertain if sleep deprivation does occur in selected postoperative open-heart surgical patients; to determine the amount of uninterrupted rest apparently available to patients; to learn if behavioral manifestations indicative of sleep deprivation occur; and to determine the nature of nursing measures which may interfere with patients' sleep (p. 348).

The method used to collect data was the descriptive survey, in which Woods employed preoperative interviews regarding previous sleep patterns, nonparticipant observation postoperatively, and terminal interviews with patients. The findings, conclusions, and recommendations she made appear to be consistent with the purposes and the data analysis, and relate to numbers and types of interruptions and to nursing measures which may help or hinder the patient in obtaining uninterrupted sleep.

SERENDIPITOUS FINDINGS

No discussion of findings would be complete without at least a brief mention of the role of serendipity in research. One occasionally hears of valuable findings which appear to occur spontaneously while the investigator is carrying out a study related to something else. The trained, experienced observer is likely to recognize a serendipitous finding when it presents itself, but the novice may pass it over. The moral appears to be that if something in the study keeps "bugging" you, take time out to examine it—you may have found another study in the making, or you may have made a discovery more important than any inherent in the purpose of your study.

SUMMARY

In concluding this chapter, we suggest that you review the findings, conclusions, and recommendations of other studies in the literature. Look particularly to see whether they are consistent with the purpose, hypothesis, method of collecting data, and analysis of the data. Note also whether limitations of the study are recognized and taken into account in the conclusions reached.

REFERENCES

Brink, Pamela J. Behavioral characteristics of heroin addicts on a short-term detoxification program. *Nurs Res* 21:38–45, Jan.-Feb. 1972.

Eisler, Jeanne; Wolfer, John A.; and Diers, Donna. Relationship between need for social approval and postoperative recovery and welfare. *Nurs Res* 21:520–525, Nov.-Dec. 1972.

Elms, Roslyn R. Recovery room behavior and postoperative convalescence. *Nurs Res* 21:390–397, Sept.-Oct. 1972.

Walker, Betty Boyd. The postsurgery heart patient: amount of uninterrupted time for sleep and rest during the first, second, and third postoperative days in a teaching hospital. *Nurs Res* 21:164–169, Mar.-Apr. 1972.

Woods, Nancy Fungate. Patterns of sleep in postcardiotomy patients. *Nurs Res* 21:347–352, July-Aug. 1972.

10

THE RESEARCH REPORT: COMMUNICATING THE FINDINGS

One final task remains to be done after a study is completed—the writing of the research report. When a study has been carried out meticulously and careful records were kept as the study progressed, all material needed for the report should be at hand. This will include a statement of the problem, the literature review that provided the documentation or rationale and background for the study, the statement of questions to be examined or the hypotheses, the collected data, the data analysis, and the conclusions that have been drawn and further questions that have been raised.

Remember that the purpose of a research report is to communicate what was done in the study to the particular individuals interested in the topic of your study. Communication of nursing research must be carried out for two groups of people—other investigators and consumers of research. Other investigators need to be aware of your research as it relates to their own efforts; they may be interested in replicating your research or building on it and thus extending its value. Consumers of research need to know about your research if it is to make a difference in nursing practice.

A research report is intended to be informative, not entertaining. However, it should be well organized and written in a readable style using clear, simple language. Technical phrases and words should be used only when they are clearly needed. Before you start to write you may wish to consult a few references on writing. Appendix A (p. 121) contains a list of books on style and writing which might be helpful. You will also want to have a good, up-to-date dictionary at hand while you are writing.

If you find it difficult to get started on writing your report, you are no different from many persons when they sit down to write. However, there is only one way to handle this problem and that is to put pencil to paper. Since the organization of the report is very important in presenting your material well, you should probably start by making a tentative outline. The entries in the outline may very well become the various subheadings of your report. The next step is to compose the first paragraph of the first section. One way to start this paragraph is to make a simple statement of the problem studied. You may want to change this introduction later, but at the moment you need to get off the ground.

For the most part, research reports are written in the past tense. The authors cited in your literature review have written in the past, your study was conducted in the past, and your study findings have also been stated in the past. The present tense may be used, however, in reports and discussions of hypotheses and theories which are broadly accepted at the present time. The future tense is rarely used in research reports except for making recommendations or for extrapolating implications for nursing when this is appropriate.

Reports should always be written objectively; that is, the personal pronoun "I" (or "we") should be reserved for the very rare occasions when the writer needs to refer to something specific about himself. Otherwise, the term "the investigator" is considered the correct one to use when referring to the person who conducted the research. The use of the passive voice may sometimes be necessary but it can easily be overdone to the extent that phrasing becomes awkward. Simply reporting, in the active voice, what was done should help to avoid this kind of awkwardness. It may be helpful for you to examine a few reports in the literature to see how other investigators have handled this aspect of their studies. You will find good as well as poor examples of writing; the former will help you know what to do and the latter may point out what to avoid.

ORGANIZING THE REPORT

Unlike other forms of writing, scientific reports (with few exceptions) usually follow a rather standardized format. An outline for a nursing research report might look something like this:

Introduction
    Statement of the problem with a brief discussion of
       its significance
    Review of the literature pertinent to the problem
       studied
    Hypotheses made or questions raised for study
Method
    Design for the study—detailed
    Study method
    Description of the sample

Description of the instruments
Description of the data analysis met
Findings
    Objective presentation of the summai
      collected
    Tables, graphs, and other illustrations as
    Results of all tests of significance or other statistical
      measures
Discussion
    Conclusions
    Interpretation of findings
    Comparison of findings with those of other investigators, if pertinent
    Implications for nursing and/or further study
Summary
    Brief statement of the problem
    Statement of the method used, findings, conclusions, and implications
References
    All references cited in the report
Appendixes
    Copies of the instruments used (questionnaires, sample forms, etc.)

The sections of the report should present objective, straightforward accounts of what was done in each step of the study. The opinions of the investigator have no place in a research report—with one exception; that is, the investigator may wish to discuss the meaning of the findings or their implications for nursing. In such a case, the departure from the report and any statements based on the investigator's own interpretation of the data should be clearly indicated.

It is also important that the investigator relate the findings to both the purpose and the limitations of the study. For example, if the study sample was small, the significance of this should be recognized; or, if the investigator did all the interviewing and recognized the existence of bias in herself, this too should be pointed out.

In the discussions of the data analysis and of the results of the study, it may be appropriate to include tables or graphs when these can show the data better, more clearly, or more dramatically than can be done by description in the text. Such "summary" tables assist in interpreting the data by displaying it in various ways. (Examples 1 and 2 in chapter 8 show tables that present summarized data.) If unsummarized raw data (i.e., the actual tallies of data) are presented, this information belongs in an appendix. Copies of instruments used (questionnaires, form letters, etc.) are also included in the appendix.

If you are writing for a periodical, you may be asked to prepare an abstract to accompany the article. The abstract should be a very brief summary of the report.

Last, but by no means least, we should say a word about titles for reports. Titles of scientific reports should be simple, descriptive statements of the nature of the study. Cute or "breezy" titles are definitely out of place. For example, if you have made a study in which the attitudes of registered nurses and social workers toward drug addicts were compared, the title of your report might well be "Comparison of the Attitudes of Registered Nurses and Social Workers toward Drug Addicts."

The books on style and writing listed in Appendix A will prove useful, especially when one is deciding on the format for the report and the general style of writing and citing references.

WRITING FOR PUBLICATION

In addition to preparing a report of your research, you may wish to bring your study to the attention of nurses generally by writing one or more articles based on it for publication in one or more of the professional journals. Before doing so, it would be a good idea for you to look at some recent issues of these journals and note the kind and length of articles they tend to publish; the type of article you write will depend on the journal you select.

All professional journals have editorial policies regarding the subject matter of articles they accept for publication. They also have directions or specifications for the preparation of manuscripts, which they will send you upon request. When you write for these specifications, it is a good idea to inquire if the editors would be interested in an article on the subject of your study. All journals have space limitations, and if the journal you select has recently carried articles similar to yours, it may not be interested in publishing another one until considerable time has elapsed. In that case, you can query another journal which might be interested. Today, nurse authors have a rather wide range of professional journals to choose from. (Consult the *International Nursing Index* under "Publications Indexed" for a list of nursing journals.)

If the journal you select expresses interest in your article, follow their style in preparing it. Send the editor the number of copies required and be sure to keep a copy for yourself. Do not use erasable paper ("corrasable" bond); there is too much chance of something getting rubbed off during the handling necessary for editing the article.

Many professional journals that report research—*Nursing Research,* for example—have all manuscripts that are submitted for publication reviewed by a team of volunteer experts. Other journals have manuscripts reviewed by several editors on their regular staff. In any event, the review takes time, and you may not hear about the disposition of your manuscript for three or four months. Most journals acknowledge receipt of a manuscript immediately by card or form letter, but the author probably does not hear until much later whether the material has been accepted. Following acceptance, another six months or even a year may go by before the author sees his article or report in print. Not only does the process of preparing a paper and scheduling it for publication take time, but some journals always have a number of accepted manuscripts already on hand and yours must wait its turn.

What should you do if your manuscript is declined, or if the editors of the journal you have selected suggest that you make major revisions in it? If you can make the suggested revisions, do so, and then resubmit the article. If a journal declines your paper, this does not necessarily mean that you should give up the idea of trying to get it published. As noted earlier, several journals that publish nursing articles are available to you, and rejection by one does not close the door to publication. Select another journal, find out what its requirements for articles are, look your manuscript over to make sure it meets these requirements, and send it off again. If the journal that rejected your paper gave you the reasons for its rejection, make the suggested changes or corrections before you send it to someone else, if it is possible for you to do so.

SUMMARY

Generally, research is not considered complete until it has been published, thus making results of the study available to others. One of the great needs in nursing today is for nurses generally to read and evaluate reports of research that is being done and to make use of research findings, when indicated, for the improvement of nursing practice. In this chapter we have concentrated on the importance of communicating to the nursing profession the results of research that has been done. Now we are ready to consider the important steps of evaluation and implementation of research findings.

III

EVALUATION
OF RESEARCH

11

THE EVALUATION PROCESS

For nursing research to have the greatest possible impact on nursing and the nursing process, practicing nurses must be familiar with the research that has been carried out and must be able to determine its usefulness. This is one of the most important functions of every nurse. To some it may seem a formidable task, but those who have read the previous chapters of this book already have an introduction to the basic facts about research that are needed to evaluate the studies of others.

The first question one should ask when evaluating a study should be: How much confidence can I place in the findings of the studies reported? One measure of confidence relates to the reputation of the investigator. Is she well known in the field under study? What are her qualifications for doing the research? Most research reports carry a brief statement about the author or investigator which will enable you to estimate, at least with some degree of confidence, her qualifications to do the research and the extent to which you can probably rely on her findings. Sometimes a less experienced investigator works under the guidance of a more sophisticated researcher; this should help to substantiate the quality of her work.

Another measure of quality is related to the periodical in which the report is published. Articles submitted to scientific journals are subjected to evaluation prior to publication, usually by reviewers or referees who are experts in the subject studied and the research methods used. Therefore, one can justifiably feel additional confidence in the reports these journals publish.

In addition to the two measures of quality mentioned above, nurses must also make their own decisions about the quality and significance of the research reported. Remember that most research has certain limitations. The purpose of any investigation is to search for truth. However, all research reflects the state of present knowledge and, because of this and because of the limitations in the research process itself, findings rarely include the ultimate answer. The work must be evaluated in terms of how much it enlarges present knowledge and what future investigations it suggests.

A first step in evaluation is careful reading of the report as a whole. A good report will be well organized around the usual steps in the research procedure and the information will be logically presented. With minor variations, scientific reports commonly follow the outline suggested in chapter 10. As you read, ask yourself questions about each part of the report.

THE RESEARCH PROBLEM

The first few questions you might ask are: What was the purpose of this study? Why was it done? Does the introduction clearly state the problem investigated? What was the scope of the problem? Were the limits of the study clearly indicated? One needs to have a clear understanding of the problem under investigation in order to evaluate the soundness of the method used to study it.

Your next question might be: How significant was the problem? This query, of course, relates directly to the purpose of the study. A criticism sometimes heard is that some research has no significance for nursing. For example, the value of basic research, that is, research in the basic sciences, may be questioned. Nevertheless, basic research often has long-range ultimate effects that are of great significance to nursing. Consider, for example, McKinnon-Mullett's (1972) investigation of capillary microscopy; it may result in no immediate changes in nursing care, but the far-reaching effects may be very important. On the other hand, the Verhonick et al. (1972) study of decubitus ulcers would appear to have more immediate and direct significance, since it dealt with an important aspect of patient care. It is true, though, that some research may be focused on problems that are more obviously significant than others. How well does the investigator justify her study in this regard? To answer this question, and to determine the importance of the study, will require that you bring your own judgment to the evaluation process.

THE LITERATURE REVIEW

Once you have determined the problem under study and its significance, an examination of the investigator's review of the literature is in order. How did she relate this review to the problem studied? Did it lead logically to the hypothesis or the questions raised for study? Sometimes literature reviews have little relevance to the study; the author may report a series of studies in related areas but does not tie them in with the present investigation. The literature review should help clarify the problem, identify and relate previous research in the area to this study, and lead logically to the question to be studied. It should also clearly identify the theoretical framework of the research when this is an important aspect of the study.

THE HYPOTHESIS

After you have examined the investigator's literature review, you may ask whether the hypothesis or the question to be studied is clearly stated. The research question should be one that can be studied with the research tools at hand. Hypotheses such as those stated by Lindeman (1972, p. 197) in her study "Nursing Intervention with the Presurgical Patient: Effectiveness and Efficiency of Group and Individual Preoperative Teaching—Phase Two" were clearly appropriate in that the means of collecting the necessary data were at hand.

Probably at this point you will ask: Are all terms specific to the study clearly defined in the report? In many instances, the answer to this question will be very important. (See Lindeman's [1972] operational definitions, pp. 197-198).

THE RESEARCH METHOD

When you come to the description of the research method used in a report you are evaluating, your questions probably will include: Was the method used descriptive, experimental, or historical—and was it appropriate to the problem studied and the hypothesis made? For example, the hypotheses in the Lindeman study determined the method to be used—a comparative experimental design. On the other hand, Brink's (1972) study of "Behavioral Characteristics of Heroin Addicts on a Short-Term Detoxification Program," in line with its purpose, was a descriptive survey.

DATA COLLECTING PROCEDURES

Once the method of collecting data is determined, one evaluates the appropriateness of the procedures used. These should be described in sufficient detail to permit replication of the research. How was the data collected? Was the appropriate tool used? Were the data collected by questionnaire when observation methods should have been used? Was the tool used a well-established one, or one devised for the study? Was the validity and reliability of the tool described?

Was the sample appropriate? How was it selected? Was the sample size adequate? Was investigator bias controlled in any way? Were the rights of subjects protected? Did the investigator recognize any flaws or lacks in the procedures used and the possible effects of these deficiencies on the results of her research? Deficiencies do not necessarily negate the study if they are recognized and if the estimation of their effect on the results is calculated by the investigator when she is presenting her findings. There are few perfect designs, especially in clinical research, in which the complex human situations involved often introduce hard-to-control intervening factors. The purpose in evaluating design is to determine the extent to which the deficiencies invalidate the findings: they may be so minimal that they have little or no adverse effect on the results of the study.

ANALYSIS OF THE DATA

The evaluation of the data analysis, that is, the presentation of the findings, should be in terms of the objectiveness and accuracy with which this part of the study is reported. This may become the most difficult part of the evaluation, especially if sophisticated statistical measures are used. For assistance in making this part of your evaluation, you might reread chapter 8, "Analysis of the Data."

CONCLUSIONS REACHED

In evaluating the conclusions reached by the investigator, consider how far these are justified by the findings. A common error on the part of the beginning investigator is to go beyond the findings of the study in discussing conclusions reached and the general applicability of the study findings. Personal experiences or opinions may be allowed to creep in and contaminate the objectivity of the conclusions. The experienced investigator strives for utmost objectivity, uses restraint in making observations, and expresses necessary reservations in drawing conclusions. Generalizations must not go beyond the evidence presented.

Many reports include a discussion section in which the findings are related to those of other researchers. It is here that implications for nursing, if appropriate, may be made. The investigator's opinion about the significance of her findings for nursing or for further research, properly identified as her opinion, may be included. Your evaluation of these opinions will be in terms of the appropriateness of the statements concerning the implications.

SUMMARY

While not all nurses will become involved in research as investigators or as research assistants, all do have a responsibility for making appropriate use of the findings of research in their work. This chapter has outlined briefly some of the factors in evaluating the quality of research and in estimating the value of research findings for the improvement of nursing care—a major objective of nursing research. Two additional sources, Davitz and Davitz (1967) and Fox (1958), are recommended for those who wish to do further reading on the evaluation of research reports.

REFERENCES

Brink, Pamela J. Behavioral characteristics of heroin addicts on a short-term detoxification program. *Nurs Res* 21:38–45, Jan.-Feb. 1972.

Davitz, Joel R. and Davitz, Lois Jean. *A Guide for Evaluating Research Plans in Psychology and Education.* New York, Teachers College Press, Columbia University, Teachers College, 1967 (paperback).

Fox, James H. "Criteria of Good Research." *Phi Delta Kappa* 39:284–286, March 1958.

Lindeman, Carol A. Nursing intervention with the presurgical patient: effectiveness and efficiency of group and individual preoperative teaching—phase two. *Nurs Res* 21:196–209, May-June 1972.

McKinnon-Mullett, Elizabeth L. Approaches to the study of nursing questions and the development of nursing science—Circulation research: exploring its potential in clinical nursing research. *Nurs Res* 21:494–498, Nov.-Dec. 1972.

Verhonick, Phyllis J.; Lewis, David W.; and Goller, Herbert O. Thermography in the study of decubitus ulcers. *Nurs Res* 21:233–237, May-June 1972.

APPENDIX A

USEFUL REFERENCE SOURCES ON WRITING

The Elements of Style, by William Strunk, Jr., and E. B. White. 2nd ed. New York, The Macmillan Co., 1972.

The Careful Writer: A Modern Guide to English Usage, by T. M. Bernstein. New York, Atheneum Publishers, 1965.

The Golden Book on Writing, by D. Lambuth. New York, Viking Press, 1964 (paperback).

A Manual of Style, 12th ed. Chicago, University of Chicago Press, 1969.

Publication Manual, rev. ed. Washington, D.C., The American Psychological Association, 1967 (paperback).

Manual for Writers of Term Papers, Theses, and Dissertations, by K. L. Turabian. 4th ed. Chicago, University of Chicago Press, 1973 (paperback).

Words into Type, by M. Skillin and R. Gay. 2nd ed. Englewood Cliffs, New Jersey, Prentice-Hall, 1974.

APPENDIX B

STUDIES CITED
IN THIS BOOK

Austin, Anne L. *The Woolsey Sisters of New York, 1860–1900.* Philadelphia, American Philosophical Society, 1971.

Historical research, biographical in nature. An account of the role of the Woolsey sisters of New York in nursing and nursing education during the Civil War and the period following the war. A good example of careful documentation.

Baer, Eva; Davitz, Lois J.; and Lieb, Renee. Inferences of physical pain and psychological distress. I. In relation to verbal and non-verbal patient communication. *Nurs Res* 19:388-392, Sept.-Oct. 1970.

A study that grew out of previous work by Davitz and a group of students interested in investigating nurses' inferences of suffering. (See Davitz and Pendleton, 1969.)

Barham, Virginia Z. Identifying effective behavior of the nursing instructor through critical incidents. *Nurs Res* 14:65-69, Winter 1965.

A study of behavior using the critical-incident technique of collecting data.

Benner, Patricia and Kramer, Marlene. Role conceptions and integrative role behavior of nurses in special care and regular hospital nursing units. *Nurs Res* 21:20-29, Jan.-Feb. 1972.

A study of role conceptions and role behavior using a Likert-type role conception and role deprivation scale and a role behavior scale developed by one of the investigators.

Berthold, Jeanne S. Nursing research grant proposals: what influenced their approval or disapproval in two national granting agencies. *Nurs Res* 22:292-299, July-Aug. 1973.

An analysis of research grant proposals submitted to the Division of Nursing, National Institutes of Health and the American Nurses' Foundation between 1955 and August 1971. Includes an example of the use of chi-square.

Bridgman, Margaret. *Collegiate Education for Nursing*. New York, Russell Sage Foundation, 1953.

A study of nursing education in the early 1950s carried out by a nonnurse.

Brink, Pamela J. Behavioral characteristics of heroin addicts on a short-term detoxification program. *Nurs Res* 21:38-45, Jan.-Feb. 1972.

A descriptive study of the behavior of a specific type of patient. Data, mainly quantitative, were collected from the patients' records and by means of a behavioral rating scale.

Broadhurst, Jean; Rang, Geraldine G.; and Schoening, Elsa. Hand brush suggestions for visiting nurses. *Public Health Nurs* 19: 487-489, Oct. 1927.

This study of a nursing procedure is representative of nursing practice studies that were done in the 1920s and 1930s.

Brophy, Elizabeth B. Relationships among self-role congruences and nursing experience. *Nurs Res* 20:447-450, Sept.-Oct. 1971.

A study comparing real and ideal self-concepts of the nurse subjects and their perceptions of the ideal nurse role. The Hanlon Q-sort was used to collect the data.

Brown, Esther Lucile. *Nursing for the Future.* New York, Russell Sage Foundation, 1948.

A study of nursing education in the late 1940s carried out by a nonnurse.

Christy, Teresa E. Portrait of a leader: M. Adelaide Nutting. *Nurs Outlook* 17:20-24, Jan. 1969.

————. Portrait of a leader: Isabel Hampton Robb. *Nurs Outlook* 17:26-29, Mar. 1969.

————. Portrait of a leader: Lavinia Lloyd Dock. *Nurs Outlook* 17:72-75, June 1969.

————. Portrait of a leader. Isabel Maitland Stewart. *Nurs Outlook* 17:44-48, Oct. 1969.

————. Portrait of a leader: Lillian D. Wald. *Nurs Outlook* 18:50-54, Mar. 1970.

————. Portrait of a leader: Annie Warburton Goodrich. *Nurs Outlook* 18:46-50, Aug. 1970.

A series of carefully documented biographies, representative of recent historical research.

Committee on the Function of Nursing. (Eli Ginsberg, Chairman) *A Program for the Nursing Profession.* New York, Macmillan, 1948.

A study of nursing and nursing education in the late 1940s carried out by a nonnurse.

Cornell, Sudie A.; Campion, Laura; Bacero, Susan; Frazier, Judith; Kjellstrom, Mary; and Purdy, Susan. Comparison of three bowel management programs during rehabilitation of spinal cord injured patients. *Nurs Res* 22:321-328, July-Aug. 1973.

A descriptive clinical nursing study planned and carried out by a team of nurses.

Cowan, Cordelia M. A study of breast care. Part I. *Am J Nurs* 29:1165-1170, Oct. 1929; Part II *Am J Nurs* 29:1299-1306, Nov. 1929.

This study of a nursing procedure is representative of nursing practice studies in the 1920s and 1930s.

Daly, Mary McDermed and Carr, John E. Tactile contact: a measure of therapeutic progress. *Nurs Res* 16:16-21, Winter 1967.

A brief case study of one disturbed child's behavior over a period of nine sessions. The purpose of the study was to develop a tool to measure tactile contacts and to assess changes of a nonverbal nature in a child's sense of trust.

Dammann, Gloria L. A. Interprofessional aspects of nursing and social work curricula. *Nurs Res* 21:160-163, Mar.-Apr. 1972.

A questionnaire survey of schools of nursing and social work to determine the extent to which nurses and social workers at the college level learn of each other's disciplines.

Davitz, Lois Jean. Identification of stressful situations in a Nigerian school of nursing. *Nurs Res* 21:352-357, July-Aug. 1972.

A study of nursing students' identification of stressful situations during their nursing education program. Utilized the critical incident technique to collect the data. Content analysis was employed in analyzing the data.

————— and Pendleton, Sidney H. Nurses' inferences of suffering. *Nurs Res* 18:100-107, Mar.-Apr. 1969.

Report of an investigation of four aspects that influence nurses' inferences of suffering: (1) cultural differences, (2) clinical specialty, (3) patient diagnosis, and (4) patient characteristics. The investigation raised questions for further study.

Dawson, Norma and Stern, Martha. Perceptions of priorities for home nursing care. *Nurs Res* 22:145-148, Mar.-Apr. 1973.

A comparative survey of concepts held by nurses working in hospitals and those held by nurses working in community health agencies.

Dock, Lavina L. *A History of Nursing.* Vols. 3 and 4. New York, Putnam, 1912.

Historical or documentary research in the form of a history of nursing.

———— and Stewart, Isabel M. *A Short History of Nursing.* New York, Putnam, 1920.

Historical or documentary research in the form of a history of nursing.

Eisler, Jeanne; Wolfer, John A.; and Diers, Donna. Relationship between need for social approval and postoperative recovery and welfare. *Nurs Res* 21:520-525, Nov.-Dec. 1972.

A study to determine whether patients' need for social approval, as measured by a social desirability scale, is related to self-ratings of postoperative physical recovery and emotional state. Possible limitations of the social desirability scale and implications for further research are discussed.

Elms, Roslyn R. Recovery-room behavior and postoperative convalescence. *Nurs Res* 21:390-397, Sept.-Oct. 1972.

A descriptive study of recovery room behavior to determine its possible association with adaptation to surgery during hospitalization (later postoperative convalescence). Limitations of the study are considered in the discussion of findings.

Georgopoulos, Basil S. and Jackson, Marjorie M. Nursing Kardex behavior in an experimental study of patient units with and without clinical nurse specialists. *Nurs Res* 19:196-218, May-June 1970.

A major field experiment designed to study the effectiveness of the use of clinical nurse specialists. Basil Georgopoulis, Ph.D., was the principal investigator and Mrs. Jackson, a nurse, was a research assistant for the project.

Glass, Leah. *Nursing Research* abstracts: a users' study. *Nurs Res* 20:152-158, Mar.-Apr. 1971.

A questionnaire survey using a representative national sample of nurses most likely to be readers of abstracts published in *Nursing Research*.

Golub, Sharon and Resnikoff, Marvin. Attitudes toward death: a comparison of nursing students and graduate nurses. *Nurs Res* 20:503-508, Nov.-Dec. 1971.

A study to show the influence of education and experience on the attitudes toward death held by student nurses and graduate nurses and to compare these attitudes. A cross-sectional survey was made of samples of both groups; data were collected by a multiple-choice questionnaire.

Goostray, Stella. *Memoirs: Half a Century in Nursing.* Boston, Nursing Archive, Mugar Memorial Library, Boston University, 1969.

A historical or documentary study which is autobiographical in nature.

Graffam, Shirley R. Nurse response to the patient in distress—development of an instrument. *Nurs Res* 19:331-336, July-Aug. 1970.

A study made for the purpose of testing a checklist to be used in research on nurses' responses to patients' complaints of distress. Reliability, face validity, comprehensiveness, and practicality of the instrument were determined.

Katz, Violet. Auditory stimulation and developmental behavior in the premature infant. *Nurs Res* 20:196-201, May-June, 1971.

A clinical investigation made to determine whether premature infants having maternal auditory stimulation will show greater maturation and greater auditory and visual function than those not having this stimulation. Tape recordings of the mother's voice were used for five minutes, six times a day, at two-hour intervals from the fifth day of life until the normal gestational age was reached.

Kellberg, Elsa R. Coronary care nurse profile. *Nurs Res* 21:30-37, Jan.-Feb. 1972.

A questionnaire was used to interview nurses via a telephone lecture network system for the purpose of comparing attitudes about nursing among those working in coronary care units with those working in other hospital units.

Kolthoff, Norma J. Microcirculation in human skin. In *American Nurses' Association Eighth Nursing Research Conference,* Albuquerque, New Mexico, March 15-17, 1972. New York, The Association, 1972, pp. 87-100.

Physiological research—an example of basic research carried out by a nurse-physiologist.

Lenburg, Carrie B.; Burnside, Helen; and Davitz, Lois J. Inferences of physical pain and psychological distress. III. In relation to length of time in the nursing education program. *Nurs Res* 19:399-401, Sept.-Oct. 1970.

A study that grew out of previous work by Davitz and a group of students interested in investigating nurses' inferences of suffering. (See Davitz and Pendleton, 1969.)

———— ; Glass, Helen P.; and Davitz, Lois J. Inferences of physical pain and psychological distress. II. In relation to the stage of the patient's illness and occupation of the perceiver. *Nurs Res* 19:392-398, Sept.-Oct. 1970.

A study that grew out of previous work by Davitz and a group of students interested in investigating nurses' inferences of suffering. (See Davitz and Pendleton, 1969.)

Lindeman, Carol A. Nursing intervention with the presurgical patient: effectiveness and efficiency of group and individual preoperative teaching—Phase II. *Nurs Res* 21:196-209, May-June 1972.

A clinical nursing study, experimental in type. A comparative study of the effect of individual and group preoperative teaching, the subjects for each type of teaching being randomly assigned.

———— and Van Aernam, Betty. Nursing Intervention with the presurgical patient—the effects of structured and unstructured preoperative teaching. *Nurs Res* 20:319-332, July-Aug. 1971.

A comparative study of the effects of two types of preoperative teaching. A good example of the relationship between the hypotheses and the design of the study. Also, it shows how nursing practitioners can become involved in the research.

MacCarthy, Jessie and Morison, Joan. An explanatory test of a method of studying illness among preschool children. *Nurs Res* 21:319-326, July-Aug. 1972.

A questionnaire study of the incidence of illness among pre-school children testing a method of studying clustering of illness within families. The method tested was not recommended for studying illness clustering in families.

Mansfield, Louise W. The use of electrocardiographic monitoring in nursing research. In *American Nurses' Association Second Nursing Research Conference,* Phoenix, Arizona, February 28, March 1-2, 1966. New York, The Association, 1966.

A descriptive study of the effects of various physical and nursing care activities on subjects' electrocardiograms. Observations were made using electrocardiographic monitoring.

Marshall, Jon C. and Feeney, Sally. Structured versus intuitive intake interview. *Nurs Res* 21:269-272, May-June 1972.

A descriptive nursing study that compared two methods of doing a specific nursing procedure.

McBride, Mary Angela B. Nursing approach, pain and relief: an exploratory experiment. *Nurs Res* 16:337-341, Fall 1967.

A clinical experiment based on the assumption that a nursing approach that assessed the psychosomatic character of the patient's pain by exploring with him the meaning of his verbal and nonverbal behavior would be followed by more appropriate nursing intervention than if his pain medication were automatically given.

Mckinnon-Mullett, Elizabeth L. Approaches to the study of nursing questions and the development of nursing science. Circulation research: exploring its potential in clinical nursing research. *Nurs Res* 21:494-498, Nov.-Dec. 1972.

Physiological research—an example of basic research carried out by a nurse-physiologist. A discussion of the potential contribution of basic research to clinical nursing research.

Monteiro, Lois. Research into things past: tracking down one of Miss Nightingale's correspondents. *Nurs Res* 21:526-529, Nov.-Dec. 1972.

Historical or documentary research that demonstrated one method of searching for documentation of historical materials—in this instance, letters.

Nichols, Glennadee A.; Kucha, Deloros H.; and Mahoney, Rosemarie F. Rectal thermometer placement times for febrile adults. *Nurs Res* 21:76-77, Jan.-Feb. 1972.

A study to determine optimum times for rectal thermometer placement for febrile adults.

———; Kulvi, Ruth L.; Life, Hazel R.; and Christ, Nancy M. Measuring oral and rectal temperatures of febrile children. *Nurs Res* 21:261-264, May-June 1972.

A study to determine optimum times for oral and rectal thermometer placement for febrile children.

Nutting, M. Adelaide. The education and professional position of nurses. In *Report of the Commissioner of Education for the Year Ending June 30, 1906*. Washington, D.C., Government Printing Office, 1907, pp. 155-205.

A very early, probably the earliest, important study of nursing education in the United States by an American nurse.

——— and Dock, Lavinia L. *A History of Nursing*. Vols. 1 and 2. New York, Putnam, 1907.

Historical or documentary research in the form of a history of nursing.

Parsons L. Claire. The effect of stimulation of the "nonspecific region of the thalamus" upon the intracellular activity of neurons in the motor cortex made epileptic with strychnine. In *American Nurses' Association Eighth Nursing Research Conference,* Albuquerque, New Mexico, March 15-17, 1972. New York, The Association, 1972, pp. 101-112.

Physiological research—an example of basic research carried out by a nurse-physiologist.

Porter, Luz S. The impact of physical-physiological activity on infants' growth and development. *Nurs Res* 21:210-219, May-June 1972.

A clinical nursing study experimental in type. Subjects were matched and randomly assigned to either a control or experimental group: the experimental group received a planned exercise regimen. Illustrative of studies that utilize a theoretical framework.

Richards, Mary Ann Bruegel. A study of differences in psychological characteristics of students graduating from three types of basic nursing programs. *Nurs Res* 21:258-261, May-June 1972.

A study to determine psychological differences among graduates of three types of basic nursing education programs using an intelligence test, a personality inventory, and a professionalization scale.

Roberts, Mary M. *American Nursing: History and Interpretation.* New York, Macmillan Company, 1954.

A history of American nursing that illustrates careful documentation and interpretation.

Ross, S. Ann. Infusion phlebitis: selected factors. *Nurs Res* 21: 313-318, July-Aug. 1972.

A clinical nursing study, exploratory and descriptive in type.

Possible relationships between five factors and the incidence of phlebitis in continuous intravenous infusions were studied.

Ryan, Elizabeth and Miller, Virginia B. Disinfection of clinical thermometers. *Am J Nurs* 32:197-206, Feb. 1932.

An example of nursing procedure studies done in the 1920s and 1930s.

Segall, Mary E. Cardiac responsivity to auditory stimulation in premature infants. *Nurs Res* 21:15-19, Jan.-Feb. 1972.

An experimental clinical nursing study in which data were collected by means of electrocardiograms and beat-by-beat cardiotachometry.

Stewart, Isabel M. and Austin, Anne L. *A History of Nursing.* New York, Putnam, 1962.

Historical or documentary research in the form of a history of nursing.

Valadez, Ana M. and Anderson, Elizabeth T. Rehabilitation workshops: change in attitudes in nurses. *Nurs Res* 21:132-137, Mar.-Apr. 1972.

A study of attitude change using a one-group pretest-posttest design.

Verhonick, Phyllis J.; Lewis, David W.; and Goller, Herbert O. Thermography in the study of decubitus ulcers. *Nurs Res* 21: 233-237, May-June 1972.

A description of a new method for studying the relationship between pressure and temperature for the purpose of comparing high-risk and nonhigh-risk patients with regard to susceptibility to decubitus ulcers.

———— ; Nichols, Glennadee A.; Glor, Beverly A.K.; and Mc-

Carthy, Rosemary T. I came, I saw, I responded: nursing observation and action survey. *Nurs Res* 17:38-44, Jan.-Feb. 1968.

A descriptive survey made for the purpose of analyzing types of responses made by professional nurses to specific nursing situations. The responses were analyzed in terms of the relevant observations made by the nurses by level of academic degree held. Filmed sequences of typical patient situations were shown using rear-view projectors. A total of 1,576 subjects viewed one of the sequences and wrote their observations and responses to the situation on data collection cards. They included biographical data on the same cards.

Walker, Betty Boyd. The postsurgery heart patient: amount of uninterrupted time for sleep and rest during the first, second, and third preoperative days in a teaching hospital. *Nurs Res* 21:164-169, Mar.-Apr. 1972.

A descriptive study based on careful clinical observations by the investigator using a data recording sheet. Limitations of the study are recognized and recommendations for additional studies are made. Implications for nursing are also discussed.

Wasserberg, Chelly and Northam, Ethel. Some time studies in obstetrical nursing. *Am J Nurs* 27:543-544, July 1927.

A brief report of two time studies that are representative of such studies done in the 1920s and 1930s.

Waters, Verle H.; Chater, Shirley S.; Vivier, Mary L.; Urrea, Judith H.; and Wilson, Holly S. Technical and professional nursing: an exploratory study. *Nurs Res* 21:124-131, Mar.-Apr. 1972.

A descriptive study of technical and professional nursing practice in the clinical setting. Observation and interview methods were used. Nurses observed were informed of the purpose to study decision making, but were not told that this would be analyzed in terms of whether this activity was technical or professional in nature, since this information might have affected their actions during the study.

Wheeler, Claribel A. (Ed.) A study of the nursing care of tuberculosis patients. *Am J Nurs* 38:1021-1037, Sept. 1938.

A three-month study of nursing routines as carried on in six hospitals to determine what constituted good nursing practice in the care of tuberculosis patients. Representative of nursing care studies done during the 1930s.

White, Marguerite B. Importance of selected nursing activities. *Nurs Res* 21:4-14, Jan.-Feb. 1972.

A comparison of responses of hospitalized adults and professional nurses on a checklist of selected nursing activities. Each activity was rated on a six-point scale from "extreme importance" to "does not apply."

Wilcox, Jane. Observer factors in the measurement of blood pressure. *Nurs Res* 10:4-17, Winter 1961.

In this investigation inter-observer variability of graduate nurses measuring blood pressure was observed. Variability was found in reading the systolic and the phase 4 and phase 5 diastolic levels. This variability was not related to selected personality or occupational factors.

Williams, Anne. A study of factors contributing to skin breakdown. *Nurs Res* 21:238-343, May-June 1972.

A longitudinal descriptive study of a clinical nursing problem—decubitus ulcers. Data were obtained by observing patients over a period of time and rating the condition of the skin.

Woodham-Smith, Cecil. *Florence Nightingale.* New York, McGraw-Hill, 1951.

Historical or documentary research which is biographical in nature.

Woods, Nancy Fungate. Patterns of sleep in postcardiotomy patients. *Nurs Res* 21:347-352, July-Aug. 1972.

A descriptive study using nonparticipant observation to collect naturalistic data in the sequence of their occurrence. The investigator pointed out the limitations of the study prior to presenting the findings.

GLOSSARY
OF SELECTED
RESEARCH TERMS

applied research seeks to find solutions to practical problems; for example, clinical research on problems in nursing practice. See **research**.

assumptions facts generally accepted as true or correct.

basic research research that seeks to advance scientific knowledge by establishing new knowledge or facts and developing fundamental theories or principles. The findings of basic research may not be immediately applicable in the solution of problems, but may lead to further research. Also called **pure research**. See **research**.

case study an in-depth study involving only one subject; occasionally used in nursing research.

chi-square (x^2) a statistical test of significance of data obtained. It is the sum of the quotients obtained by dividing the square of the differences between the observed and theoretical or expected frequencies by the theoretical frequencies.

content analysis categories appropriate subject headings or classifications that an investigator establishes for the purpose of organizing data collected in a study.

139

content validity   validity of a data collecting instrument that is established by pointing out the authority for the items used in a questionnaire or checklist.

control variable   a factor in a study that is held constant so as not to intervene and influence the results; for example, age or income of the subjects or type of surgery performed on them. See **variable.**

correlation   a measure of degree of relationship between the variables studied. The computed values fall between a $+1$ and -1. The closer to $+1$ or -1 they fall the higher will be the degree of relationship or correlation of the variables.

correlational survey   a survey used to collect data from a group on two or more variables to estimate the relationship between the variables.

criterion measure   a characteristic quality or attribute used to measure the effect of an independent variable upon the subjects under study.

criterion variable   see **dependent variable.**

critical incident technique   a method of obtaining data from study subjects' written reports of previous experiences or incidents in their lives which are related to the matter under study.

cross-sectional survey   a survey used to collect comparative data on two or more groups at the same point in time but at different points in the experience of the groups.

data   facts or phenomena. In research the term commonly refers to the facts observed or obtained in some other way (singular-datum).

deductive reasoning the development of logical answers or conclusions from reliable premises. It starts with general propositions and uses these to derive conclusions; i.e., it goes from the general to the particular.

dependent variable the variable under observation by the investigator who wishes to note the effect on it of the introduction of an independent variable. Sometimes called the **criterion variable**.

descriptive research present-oriented research that seeks to accurately describe what *is* and to analyze the facts obtained in relation to the problem under study. It may lead to theories or hypotheses to be tested experimentally.

documentary research see **historical research**.

empirical name given to a method of testing or verifying a hypothesis by means of observation or experience. In empirical research the observations are systematically controlled.

experimental research future-oriented research that tests a hypothesis or hypotheses by setting up a controlled situation and then manipulating it to determine the effect of the manipulation. The design for experimental research consists in control and experimental groups which are tested before and after the manipulation of the experimental group or groups. Also called **explanatory research.**

exploratory study a preliminary study designed to help refine the problem, develop or refine hypotheses, or test and refine the data collecting methods. Also called **pilot study.**

external criticism investigation to determine whether data collected for a study is what it purports to be (authorship, date, etc.).

face validity validity of a data collecting instrument that is assumed after simple inspection of the items on a questionnaire or checklist.

forced-choice arrangement see **Q-sort technique.**

frequencies or **frequency distribution** a way of ordering data to show the number of subjects for each value or score in a study.

historical research past-oriented research that seeks facts that will help one to interpret and understand past events and their influences. The method used is systematic documentation of the evidence and evaluation of its authenticity.

hypothesis a statement of predicted relationships between the factors, or variables, under study. It is the tentative deduction usually made as a first step in research (hypotheses–plural).

independent variable the variable the investigator manipulates or introduces into the situation. Sometimes called the **manipulated variable.**

inductive reasoning the development of logical answers or generalizations by explaining relationships based on facts obtained through observation. Starts with particular situations and goes to general propositions.

internal criticism investigation to determine the accuracy of statements in authenticated data that have been collected for a historical study.

interval data data representing points on a scale; e.g., body temperature readings.

interview a method of collecting data by means of verbal questioning.

level of significance refers to the probability that differences between sets of data are due to chance.

logic a method of reasoning: a science involved in the development of principles governing inference.

longitudinal survey a survey that collects data over a period of time for use in studying changes that occur as a result of the experiences occurring or introduced during a specified time period. Also called **prospective study**.

manipulated variable see **independent variable.**

mean the score obtained by adding all the scores or values and dividing this sum by the total number of scores or values: a measure of central tendency.

median the exact middle score or value in a distribution of scores; obtained by separating the scores or values into an upper and lower half: a measure of central tendency.

mode the score or value that occurs most frequently in a distribution of scores or values: a measure of central tendency.

nominal data data that consist of names of things or conditions (age, sex, race, diagnosis).

normal curve a bell-shaped curve showing how values or scores cluster. In a normal distribution approximately 68 percent of all scores will fall between a $+1$ and a -1 standard deviation; approximately 95 percent will fall between $+2$ and -2 standard deviations; almost all will fall between $+3$ and -3 standard deviations.

null hypothesis a hypothesis which predicts that there will be no significant differences between the results of measures testing control and experimental groups following manipulation of the experimental group. It is related to the statistical test to be used. Rejection of the null hypothesis indicates that there is a statistically significant difference (or differences) between the groups examined.

observation   a method of collecting data by means of one or more persons who observe and record the activity or behavior being studied.

opinionaire   see **questionnaire**.

ordinal data   data which consists of numbers (e.g., of subjects involved) or rank order (e.g., rankings of patient behaviors).

pilot study   see **exploratory study**.

primary source   a data source that provides direct evidence of an actual event. May be published or unpublished. Examples: the letters of an individual whose life is being studied; an actual tape recording of a meeting.

proposition   a term used in logic to indicate a statement that characterizes something as true or false.

prospective study   see **longitudinal survey**.

Q-sort technique   a method of obtaining data about attitudes: a forced-choice method of rating. Subjects sort cards into a specified number of piles according to the rating the subject gives the object or behavior listed on the card. The number of cards that can be placed in each pile creates an arrangement similar to the normal curve.

questionnaire   a paper and pencil method of gathering data from subjects in a study. Data sought usually involve the knowledge, attitudes, observations, or experiences of the subjects. When opinions are sought, the instrument used may be called an opinionaire.

random sample a sample in which everyone in the group to be sampled has an equal chance or probability to be selected.

range the distance between the top and bottom scores or values in a distribution of scores or values.

reliability refers to the accuracy of the data collection instrument with respect to stability and repeatability. The instrument should be capable of obtaining consistent results when reused.

research a systematic inquiry to discover facts or test theories in order to obtain valid answers to questions raised or solutions for problems identified.

sample a selection of individuals from the total population of a particular class of individuals. For example, the selection of a group of registered nurses in one state in the United States from the total population of registered nurses in that state.

scientific method a systematic method employed in study or research in which a problem is identified, a hypothesis (or hypotheses) is made, and data are gathered, systematically arranged, and interpreted in order to empirically test the hypothesis.

secondary source a data source that is one or more steps removed from the actual event described. A history of an event may contain material from primary sources but it is itself a secondary source.

standard deviation a measure of the variability of scores or values about the mean.

standard error   an estimate of sampling error using a statistical formula. It is an estimate of the normal distribution of all the means that would be obtained if the study were replicated using all samples in the population under study. The standard error of the mean can be obtained by dividing the standard deviation of the mean of the sample by the square root of the number in the sample.

statistical inference   a method of statistical analysis used to enable one to make inferences about data; i.e., to determine whether differences between sets of data are significant and to make generalizations which can apply to larger populations.

stratified random sample   a sample that has been randomized according to some added factor(s) (age, religious affiliation, etc.). See **sample, random sample.**

structured interview   an interview that follows a set pattern of questioning; used for obtaining more objective data than can be obtained when open-end questions are used.

symbols   are frequently used in research. Some commonly used are:

r correlation	$>$ greater than
p probability	x^2 chi-square
$<$ less than	Σ sum

tests of significance   statistical methods of determining whether an observed difference in two sets of data is small and therefore not significant, or large and therefore significant.

theoretical framework   provides the theoretical approach to an investigation. The hypothesis and design of the research will be related to the theory selected.

theory   an explanation of facts, or a set of propositions, used as principles to explain a particular class of phenomena.

t **test** a statistical test of significance to determine differences between means of small, randomly selected samples. *t* is equal to the difference between sample and population means divided by the standard error of the difference in sample means.

unstructured interview an interview that utilizes open-end questions to obtain freer responses than can be obtained when a set pattern of questioning is followed.

validity refers to the ability of a data collection method or other instrument to obtain the relevant needed data or to measure what it is supposed to measure.

variable any factor, characteristic, quality, or attribute under study.